HOW TO
OVERCOME
"COOL DOWN"
AND
KEEP THE FIRE BURNING

by Charles ♥ *Frances Hunter*
and Ralph Turner

Published by HUNTER BOOKS
201 McClellan Road
Kingwood, Texas 77339, U.S.A.

BOOKS BY CHARLES ♥ FRANCES HUNTER

A CONFESSION A DAY KEEPS THE DEVIL AWAY
ANGELS ON ASSIGNMENT
ARE YOU TIRED?
BORN AGAIN! WHAT DO YOU MEAN?
COME ALIVE
DON'T LIMIT GOD
FOLLOW ME
GO, MAN, GO
GOD IS FABULOUS
GOD'S ANSWER TO FAT...LOØSE IT!
GOD'S CONDITIONS FOR PROSPERITY
HANDBOOK FOR HEALING
HANG LOOSE WITH JESUS
HIS POWER THROUGH YOU
HOT LINE TO HEAVEN
HOW DO YOU TREAT MY SON JESUS?
HOW TO HEAL THE SICK
HOW TO MAKE YOUR MARRIAGE EXCITING
HOW TO OVERCOME "COOL DOWN" AND KEEP THE FIRE BURNING
How to Receive and Minister THE BAPTISM WITH THE HOLY SPIRIT
I DON'T FOLLOW SIGNS AND WONDERS...THEY FOLLOW ME!
IF YOU REALLY LOVE ME...
IMPOSSIBLE MIRACLES
MEMORIZING MADE EASY
MY LOVE AFFAIR WITH CHARLES
NUGGETS OF TRUTH
POSSESSING THE MIND OF CHRIST
P.T.L.A. (Praise the Lord, Anyway!)
SINCE JESUS PASSED BY
the fabulous SKINNIE MINNIE RECIPE BOOK
STRENGTH FOR TODAY
SUPERNATURAL HORIZONS (from Glory to Glory)
THE TWO SIDES OF A COIN
THIS WAY UP!
VIDEO STUDY GUIDE - HOW TO HEAL THE SICK (14 Hours)
VIDEO STUDY GUIDE - HOW TO HEAL
THE SICK POWER PACK (6 Hours)
VIDEO STUDY GUIDE - THE BOOK OF ACTS (6 Hours)
WHY SHOULD "I" SPEAK IN TONGUES???

©Copyright 1990 by Charles and Frances Hunter, all rights reserved. Printed in U.S.A.
Published by HUNTER BOOKS, 201 McClellan Road, Kingwood, Texas 77339, U.S.A.

ISBN # 1-878209-02-7

©Scripture quotations are taken from:
The Authorized King James Version (KJV).
The New King James Version (NKJV), ©1979, 1980, 1982, 1983 by Thomas Nelson, Inc.,
Nashville, Tn.
The Amplified New Testament (Amp.), ©The Lockman Foundation 1954, 1958.
New American Standard Bible, ©The Lockman Foundation, 1960, 1962, 1963, 1968, 1971,
1972, 1973, 1975, 1977.

TABLE OF CONTENTS

For other information about the GCA or video/audio tapes and books,
price lists, and order forms, write to:
Charles and Frances Hunter
201 McClellan Road
Kingwood, Texas 77339, U.S.A.
Telephone (713) 358-7575

For information about Charles and Frances Hunter's Healing Explosions, video teaching tapes, audio tapes, and books, foreign languages for missions training and Great Commission Army write to:

Charles ♥ Frances Hunter
201 McClellan Road
Kingwood, Texas 77339, U.S.A.

INTRODUCTION

Every pastor who is called of God and given by Jesus Christ to the local church has the God-given desire in his heart to extend the Kingdom of God on earth. Emphasis may differ and the approach may vary, but the desire is the same — to get the gospel of Jesus Christ into the hearts of men that they may be delivered from the power of darkness. Every pastor who is a man of God should welcome every attempt to aid him in involving the people in the work of evangelizing the world.

God has placed in the hearts of Charles and Frances Hunter the vision for a Great Commission Army with hundreds of thousands of enthusiastic believers witnessing the gospel everywhere, on the job, in the market places, on the streets, in airports, in the community where they live, in homes, etc., while they go about their daily lives. This witnessing will be accompanied by signs following as people are healed and delivered from the power of the demons.

The Great Commission Army is not to

be thought of as something in addition to or alongside of the church. The Church of God is the "Great Commission Army". The church, through lack of knowledge or neglect, may not be functioning as Jesus intended, but He commissioned the church at the beginning to "go into all the world and preach the gospel — baptizing, teaching, healing the sick and casting out demons."

The Great Commission Army concept is a plan to train, motivate and mobilize the people of the local church to function as the army of God. God will raise up His army in these last days. This Great Commission Army is not a threat to the work of the pastor in the local church. It can be a valuable aid to him in accomplishing the work God gave him to do.

Every sincere man of God wishes to expand the kingdom of God on earth. The Great Commission Army concept can accelerate this expansion by giving the people the "How-to" and the "motivation". Getting the people involved in power evangelism will bring about growth in them as well as in church membership. This releases the pastor to fulfill his call to feed the flock of God over which the Holy Ghost has made him overseer. It will not take away...but add to!

If the goal and desire of the pastor is to increase the size of his local flock and he believes this to be a way to extend the kingdom of God, the Great Commission Army will help him accomplish this goal and fulfill this desire. If the pastor believes the flock should remain small and other churches begun, the Great Commission Army will accomplish this.

Even though the Great Commission Army is the uniting together of hundreds of thousands of believers worldwide in this great effort, it is intended to function within the local church, bringing those being saved into the church where they can be nurtured, loved and discipled.

For that reason it is imperative that pastors of local churches catch the vision, agree and cooperate with this effort by opening the door for the people to become involved in the Great Commission Army. It is important that pastors see this not as just another program for the church, but as a genuine move of God to involve His people in the work of the kingdom as He commissioned us.

The Great Commission Army is involved in the enlistment, training, motivating, and mobilization of a force of committed believers who follow the written orders of our Commander-in-Chief, in the power of the Holy Spirit, making disciples, delivering captives, healing the sick, and training them to join with us in the same task.

The term "army" is appropriate to describe this group. We have a Commander-in-Chief, combat training, equipment, and weapons. And THERE IS A WAR ON!

The war is on! Not a defensive war, nor a war for acquisition. But a war to reclaim that which was lost by the invasion of a living thief. Our Great Commander-in-Chief, by His death, burial and resurrection, has bound the strong man, rendering him powerless, and has commissioned us to go to the captives and announce to them the good news, exercising the authority of Jesus' Name to release them.

The church of Jesus Christ is to be militant because we invade the realms of darkness where the enemy imposed his kingdom of darkness, deception and lies on men created in the image of God. Warfare results as we bring light into this darkness. *("For the weapons of our warfare are not carnal, but mighty through God to the pulling down of strong holds;) casting down imaginations, and every high thing that exalteth itself against the knowledge of God, and bringing into captivity every thought to the obedience of Christ"* (2 Cor. 10:4,5 KJV).

Just as in any other army, the Great Commission Army of the Lord has divisions according to the different needs. No army is made up entirely of "foot soldiers with a rifle". Others are as important to success as the soldiers on the front lines.

(1) There is a training department. Classroom teaching imparts the concepts. In addition to the classroom instruction there is "on the field" training as those with experience team up with newer members so they can "catch" the method as they are discipled. We learn how to witness to others, cast out demons and heal the sick by seeing it done and participating in it.

(2) Every successful army must have a Department of Intelligence to spy out the enemy and discover his tactics. An intercessory prayer group continually waits before the Lord in the Spirit while engaging the enemy in spiritual combat.

(3) It is also necessary to continually re-

cruit new soldiers for the army. A group of enthusiasts who have been involved in the Great Commission Army and are seeing success are ready to go into churches which are open to Great Commission Army soldiers to stir up those member to become involved.

(4) A diplomatic corps of pastors who have seen what happens when the door is opened to this Great Commission Army are constantly going to other pastors to encourage those pastors, creating positive relationships, so these churches will be open to this concept. Once the door is open, the recruiters can go in.

(5) Every army needs a supply group. These are people with the ministry of giving who continually pour their resources into the need of the army.

(6) Special assault troops who are highly trained and successful will target certain areas for a "blitz" when the Commander-in-Chief directs. These sometime go in just before a "Healing Explosion" and sometime just after the Explosion.

(7) Every army has its strategists. This group is composed of pastors and Great Commission Army department heads. The advisory group does not enter into decision

making, but protects the directors by their continual input and support.

Bud Gardner
Pastor, Faith Outreach Center
San Antonio, Texas

FOREWORD
By Charles ♥ Frances Hunter

As the great and powerful Healing Explosions have developed and expanded into a global ministry of training believers in multitudes of languages, cultures, denominations, and nations around the world, there always loomed before us the need to keep the trained teams active in the ministry for which they had been trained.

We are always stretched beyond a normal workload in our ministry, so we knew it would be impossible for the two of us to set up a national or international work to follow up on trained team members all over the world, but we also knew God had spoken that this was a must!

Many people offered to help and do whatever we asked them to do, but that wasn't what we needed! We needed someone who could take the plan God had given us, develop it in the Spirit and then give it to us for final approval. After our approval, then that person would carry the whole responsibility under our direction, but without our having to constantly be working on the details.

When we were organizing and developing the teams for the San Antonio Healing Explosion, one person kept shining above all others with the zeal and vision to do this work. Ralph Turner came to us with his vision. We listened, we caught his vision of our vision, and God began putting the pieces together. He presented an entire plan to us from beginning to end and we knew this was exactly the man God had selected.

Out of this beginning has developed this book HOW TO OVERCOME "COOL DOWN" AND KEEP THE FIRE BURNING. We want you to catch this vision to instill into your heart the persistence of Jesus, the New Testament apostles and disciples, and our modern day disciples to never stop until Jesus' harvest of souls is complete and He returns for us!

WHO IS RALPH TURNER?

We have appointed Ralph Turner as the national GREAT COMMISSION ARMY (GCA) director. Just as none of us know how God will develop our services for Him, nor where He may lead next, we know without a doubt that Ralph has been charged with this responsibility under our direction.

He will work under HUNTER MINISTRIES. Most communications will flow from our office, 201 McClellan Road, Kingwood, Texas 77339.

We believe God will raise up all the directors under the leadership of Ralph who will implement the GCA operations in their areas, and oversee them so the giant job Jesus gave us for this last generation (we believe) will be rapidly accomplished: Keep going daily into all of our world, preaching the Gospel (leading people to Jesus), casting out devils, ministering the baptism with the Holy Spirit to others, handling the powers and poisons of Satan, the snake in the Bible, and LAYING HANDS ON THE SICK AND SEEING THEM HEALED so they will believe in Jesus and be saved!

Jesus made His plan very plain, and we are following His scriptural authority by training believers, equipping saints under the direction of pastors, for the work of the ministry of Jesus. We want to do this as far as they will allow throughout the nation and eventually throughout the world.

Ralph will be contacting multitudes, and he will need you to contact him (through our ministry) to develop this gigantic work of OVERCOMING "COOL DOWN" AND KEEPING THE FIRE BURNING in your life!

God told us some time ago, "What you must do, do it quickly."

So we say to you, "What you must do, do it quickly!"

Now, let Ralph Turner tell his vision of our vision of the vision of Jesus.

>*Sing to the Lord, O earth,*
>*Declare EACH DAY that he is the one*
>*   who saves!*
>*Show his glory to the nations!*
>*Tell everyone about his miracles.*
>*For the Lord is great, and should be*
>*   highly praised;*
>*He is to be held in awe above all gods...*

(I Chronicles 16:23-25 TLB).

"Dear friends in Rome (that's you!): *This letter is from Paul, Jesus Christ's slave, chosen to be a missionary, and sent out to preach God's Good News. This Good News was promised long ago by God's prophets in the Old Testament. It is the Good News about his Son, Jesus Christ our Lord, who came as a human baby, born into King David's royal family line; and by being raised from the dead he was proved to be the mighty Son of God, with the holy nature of God himself.*

"And now, through Christ, all the kindness of God has been poured out upon us undeserving sinners; and now he is sending us (that's you and us) *out around the world to tell all people everywhere the great things God has done for them, so that they, too, will believe and obey him.*

"And you, dear friends in Rome" (or where you live), *are among those he dearly loves; you, too, are invited by Jesus Christ to be God's very own — yes his holy people..."*

(Romans 1:1-7 TLB).

GO, MAKE DISCIPLES!

CAPTURE A VISION!

Al, Grace, Reinette and Michelle are very special folks! But — they are no more special or different than most of you reading this. Al is a Park Ranger in San Antonio, Texas. Grace works for Southwest Airlines as a booking agent. Reinette is a civilian employee at Randolph Air Force Base. She works in the civilian contract section. Michelle is a high school student. Just plain, normal folks! Just born again, Spirit-filled people.

But — *they have captured a vision!*

That is what makes them unusual! That is why their stories (in very brief form) are recorded here. They have caught the vision put forth by Charles and Frances Hunter. They have seen that not only can they "lay hands on the sick and see them recover," but that it is supposed to take place wherever they happen to be when the need is presented.

The purpose of presenting their stories here is simple! Hopefully, many of you can relate to the events given. I hope you can see that this is not only the way our lives should be lived, but it is the way you and I *can* live every day for the rest of our lives. There are very few of us who do not encounter many potential opportunities each day for ministry. What we do is stroll on by and miss those opportunities. We must learn to be attentive and obedient to the voice of the Holy Spirit as He speaks to us about those opportunities.

That is the purpose of this book! It is my prayer that the Holy Spirit will use the events and suggestions contained here to spark something inside you! I pray that spark will cause you to do whatever is necessary to ignite a flame that will burn this truth into your mind.

When our Lord said, "These signs will follow those who believe: In My Name they will cast out demons; they will speak with new tongues; they will take up serpents; and if they drink anything deadly, it will by no means hurt them; *they will lay hands on the sick, and they will recover*" (Mark 16:17,18 NKJV), Jesus was describing a continuous way of life for every believer.

To add to the excitement of reading these accounts, we have made them read like a short story. However, all the facts are actual and happened just as written. As you read them, begin to see yourself in similar situations. These actual events are certainly unique to these individuals. However, there are exciting things the Holy Spirit can provide in your life which will be every bit as dynamic.

So begin with me now a trip that I pray will result in your life becoming one continual testimony to the grace and power of our Lord Jesus Christ.

Chapter One

Al — A Cop for Jesus!

It was during the time of year that most folks in the United States have what they call winter. We call it winter in San Antonio too, but it's sure not like what we see taking place up north. Here a winter day may get down to 45 degrees. We consider that a cold day. It's that kind of day now! Clear — the sky blue with sort of a glare of white mixed in. Several vapor trails criss-cross the sky showing where planes, maybe giant bombers or planes loaded with holiday passengers, were seconds ago.

I've been patrolling in one of the many parks in San Antonio. Not much taking place today. A few persistent joggers about, now wearing their long sweats. A few even sport ski masks. And occasionally a real determined case still is wearing shorts and a long sleeved sweater. But, for the most part, today is a really quiet day.

As I drove around in the patrol car, winding through the narrow streets that carried picnickers and general park-goers to the various tabled areas, I allowed my mind to carry me back to those events that marked what was to be the beginning of the most exciting time of my life.

I remember the enthusiasm of Linda, my wife. She had begun to attend that first meeting at the church on how to heal the sick. It was the video tape course taught by Charles and Frances Hunter. I didn't know a whole lot about them, or what they did. I had only been saved about two years and I know there were a lot of things going on I didn't understand. And, besides, I had to work on the night the class was being held.

I remember those times when I would get in from patrolling my shift and Linda would have been to the Healing School. She would be almost ecstatic about what she had heard and seen that night. Things about "growing out legs and arms" and all sorts of things that sounded pretty far out. But, like I said, there were (and still are) a whole lot of things I've not even heard about yet in this Christian life.

My mind is suddenly yanked back to the present as I hear a commotion off in some trees and underbrush to my right. I pull to the edge of the grass and kill the engine. Just then four kids come running out of the brush and almost crash headlong into the side of the car. Boy, do they get wide-eyed when they have to pull up short, almost eye-ball to eye-ball with the light flasher bar on top of my patrol car. I tell them to just be careful and stay out of the brush and on the paths that zig-zag all through the park. They trot off, sheepishly laughing and waving back at me. I resume my casual patrol of the area and my mind resumes its recounting of the past few months' happenings.

Linda had told me just about everything she had learned during the class. Fourteen hours she had watched Charles and Frances Hunter give instructions on healing. There had been testimonies aplenty to verify their claims of the Power of God flowing through just "plain ol' folks". This concept had stirred something deep down inside me. It was so awesome to think that I could lay my hands on a sick person and see God's power heal them.

Linda had told me how she had been taught that healing the sick was not just a matter of praying, but it involved speaking to the illness in the Name of Jesus Christ and commanding healing to come. Wow! I'd never heard that before.

I pulled out onto one of the main streets that bordered the park and headed for the closest "Stop and Go" for a quick cup of coffee. Once again I began to recall certain life-changing events that had occurred recently. My mind zeroed in on the one event that so impacted my entire life. I can recall each detail now as though it had happened only minutes ago.

The sun had already set over San Antonio. I was on patrol at Woodlawn Lake. With the setting of the sun, the gentle breeze which had been brushing the lake into little ripples had died away. Now the only noise were the sounds of the stubborn picnickers who just refused to allow the day to draw to a close.

The lake was dead calm — and quickly disappearing to the eye as dusk passed and night was drawing its dark curtain over the trees on the far bank first. Then slowly it

moved over the lake until it began to black
out even the brush and trees close to the gate
where my partner and I had our patrol car
parked. As we sat there, each deep in his own
thought world, we were suddenly jolted
back to the present. Frantic sounds of someone telling us that a man had fallen into the
lake and drowned!

We were quickly informed that the man
had been seen going under the water some
15-20 minutes before. He pointed to the general area where the victim was last seen.

Racing to the spot, I tried to peer
through the darkness to catch a glimpse of
something — anything that might look like
someone in the water. Nothing! It was just
too dark! I began to shine my flashlight over
the top of the water.

Everything still! No movement to indi-
cate the man was still above the water.
Nothing!

Suddenly someone standing next to me
shouted that he saw something.

"Where!" I shouted!

"There!" was the reply!

I pointed my light where he indicated.
Nothing!

He took the flashlight and splashed a

beam of light to the spot where he was sure he had caught just a glimmer of something. Something under the water — just beneath the dark surface.

There! I see something — like cloth — just under the surface.

I quickly ripped off my gun belt and dove into the water. Within a matter of seconds I had reached the spot where I was sure I had seen something. As I grabbed out toward that spot, my hand closed on a shirt. Beneath the shirt — cold flesh.

Frantically I pulled upward to try to get the man's head out of the water. The water was not very deep, so I stood up and tried to locate any sign of life. NONE! Nothing! The man seemed cold and getting stiff.

Quickly my mind began to calculate. According to the witness — 20 minutes under the water by now. Maybe more! He can't be alive! Human beings just don't survive that long under water.

He is dead! No Lord! My heart cries out for his life.

Please Lord, let him be alive.

I reach the shore. My partner helps both of us out of the water. We check again. Some sign! Heartbeat! None!

Some sign that he is breathing! Just a little! None! He is dead! NO!

My partner begins CPR. No good! He isn't responding. My partner tires.

Now it's my turn! Lord, let him live!

I desperately pound on his chest trying to get his heart to beat. Nothing! I go through all the steps of CPR as I have been so well taught to do. Still, nothing! Then, from the depth of my being and up into my mind a thought comes. Right from the Spirit of God I recall something my wife had told me the Hunters had said about this kind of situation. Something about commanding life to enter — about "binding the power of death". They had even said to command the water to leave the lungs.

Could it be?

This man is dead!

Could it work?

No time to debate?

I stand with a boldness not of me and command the power of death to be bound. I command life to re-enter this man. Boldness comes with rising faith! I command in the name of Jesus for this man to return to life and lungs to empty. I can still see it as clearly as when it happened: he suddenly sits up and starts coughing mud out of his lungs.

He's alive!

It worked!

By the way, his name is Moses!

That was the most exciting time of my life! I remember the holy awe I felt some weeks later as Moses stood before the crowd at Faith Outreach Center and testified as to how God had brought him back to life and given him another chance.

It wasn't long after that when I received a call from the Chief's office. It was the voice of my boss, the police sergeant.

"Are you the one who allegedly raised a man from the dead out at Woodlawn Lake?" The shock struck me with fear, realizing that this was not a normal event for a policeman. I thought, "Oh, oh, I'm in trouble!"

"I want to see you in my office right away!"

"Yes, sir!"

A few minutes later I stood in front of the sergeant who asked me to tell him the whole story. I did, all the time wondering what his reaction would be.

His reply stunned me for a moment. He said, "I'm a Spirit-filled Christian, too. Let's form a group of Spirit-filled policemen and train them to do what God wants us to do."

As a result, a new police organization was born. We call it "Shields for Christ". We are having a monthly meeting and it is growing. We would like to see this become a national organization! We want all our members to take the video healing school training so we can know how to direct God's Holy Spirit power for his glory. Hallelujah! As I pulled into the parking slot at "Stop and Go" I gratefully think, "How great is our God." What a neat Savior we have!

The "Stop and Go" is almost deserted this time of day. I walk to the back and aim for the pot of just-made coffee. I have been here plenty of times before, so I speak to the girl manning the cash register. She nods and smiles. As I pour the hot cup of coffee and mix in the powdered cream, my mind is still being gently pulled to the recent thoughts. I feel sort of an afterglow all over just thinking about what life with Jesus Christ is like.

At the counter I pay for my coffee and glance at the girl, intending on making some positive comment that might lead into a statement about our Lord. Instead I see her wince in what seems to be pain. I ask her what is the problem? She looks at me through eyes filled with discomfort and pain and complains about the "migraine headache" that medicine doesn't seem to help.

I ask her if she knows that Jesus can heal that headache — right now?

She is plainly caught off guard at the question. She asked me if the manager put me up to that just to trick her.

I assure her that I am very serious about the question. She sees that I am! So she consents for me to pray for her. Very simply I reach across the counter and put my hand on her head. I command the headache to leave "in the name of Jesus".

It does! At once! Ha! Not only does she get healed of the headache — but as I look in amazement, she goes down under the power of God, right on the floor behind the cash register!

When she gets up she is a very surprised lady. But she is also a very overwhelmed lady. She knows she has been touched by God.

As I walk out into the bright sunlight and crisp air I cannot help but exclaim right out loud, *"How great is our God and what a neat Savior we have!"*

Chapter Two

Grace — The Airline Booking Agent

Grace has been with the airlines six years. Spending every day meeting people, most of them on the phone. Talking about their plans to travel to all sorts of places, and helping them with many of the questions for which they really need answers. It's a job that really makes her feel useful.

In the short breaks between calls she has time to reflect on the events in her life during the last year or so.

It's been some seven years now since she committed her life to Jesus Christ. What a change that made! It seemed to give everything else real meaning.

As a single parent, she and her daughter, Maureen, have grown closer and closer through the relationship both have with the Lord.

But wow! This last year has really been something else. It all began to happen last year when she enrolled in the Hunter Healing School. The announcement had mentioned that Charles and Frances would be coming to San Antonio in December to hold a giant Healing Explosion. That sounded great, but the awesome thing was that they were told that during the meeting, the people who would be praying for the sick would not be Charles and Frances, but just plain believers who were to be trained on how to heal the sick. Was it possible that she could be one of those?

It certainly seemed worth looking into.

The first session was good, hearing about the vision the Hunters had that sort of started this whole idea. They had seen the Body of Christ rising up and standing tall on the earth. Demons were seen scattering from this new wave of power and authority. And the ones doing all this were the believers — just like Grace and thousands of others — going forth and laying hands on the sick.

It was after several sessions that Grace

really began to see the impact of what was being said. The effect was so great on her that she became unsure of her salvation.

She had never laid hands on anyone and seen them healed!

She had never cast out even one demon! Yet — right there it was! Right in God's Word! *"These signs will follow those who believe: In My name they will cast out devils... they will lay hands on the sick and they will recover."*

Was she not even a believer? Slowly she began to realize that, Yes! She was born again, but she had never been told that she was supposed to be out doing these things.

If she had only known! How could she be doing these things if she had never been told? But *now she had been told!* And never again would she be satisfied with anything less. If this is what her Lord had commanded her to do, then by His grace that is exactly what she would do. It did not seem possible that God could use her that way, but if He would, then He most certainly could! So she made herself available to the Holy Spirit to be used in just whatever way He desired.

Her first opportunity had come just a short while after that commitment.

The day had been routine; a day like so many others. She had been pretty busy that morning, taking calls from folks wanting to go just about every place Southwest Airlines went, and some places she had never even heard of. Soon a break was well in order. Something to drink and a few minutes to relax would surely help.

She had gone into the ladies' lounge. At first she didn't notice her, a lady, a co-worker, standing at the sink. She was leaning on the sink, one hand on either side of it. She seemed to be looking into the bottom of the sink. Suddenly Grace was gently prompted by the Holy Spirit to approach her. Grace asked the woman what the problem was. In obvious pain, she told Grace that she was having tremendous pain in her kidneys. She had had some kidney problems and now the pain was really getting to her.

Quickly Grace "checked" in the Spirit. It was sort of a "am I on the right tract" check. Knowing that she was, she proceeded. She told the woman that she was going to place her hands on her back in the area of her kidneys, and ask Jesus to heal her. Then she commanded in the name of Jesus, that all the pain leave, and that all the parts connected with the kidneys be healed.

She picked up her purse and walked out of the ladies' room.

Grace was not to see the woman for three days. The reason was simple! Grace was about to take a three day break and just relax.

When she returned three days later, she was met by a very excited woman. The lady from the "ladies' lounge encounter" exclaimed that within 15 minutes all the pain was gone and that there had been no further problem. It has been about a year now, and there has still been no further problem.

The word spread, and others began coming to Grace for healing. She began to see that when people experience the real power of God, not just religion, they talk about it. They tell others. And many of those others want that same touch.

Yolanda was that way. Her little son had developed a very high fever and a lump on the side of his neck. Her first thought had been to get him to a doctor — quickly. The doctor had told her that unless the fever and the infection were both gone by later in the day he would have to put the child into the hospital. As she left the doctor's office, she remembered the stories being told about the lady at work who was supposed to be able to heal sick people in the name of Jesus. What if it were all true? It surely would beat a stay in the hospital! It surely would be worth a try.

She got to the office just as Grace was arriving at work. She explained the problem to her, and Grace replied by placing her hand on the lump and simply commanding the fever and the infection to leave "In Jesus' name."

The fever broke at once! Shortly afterwards the lump was gone!

Grace has been used many times since then, both at work and at church, to minister in the healing service.

One of the most interesting and exciting things happened as she, her daughter, and her mother sat down to enjoy a good meal at a local steakhouse.

As Grace was ordering her meal, all at once that gentle nudging of the Holy Spirit for which she had learned to listen became evident.

Her attention was called to a group of people sitting at a table not far away. The restaurant was crowded. It was during the noon rush. But the Lord singled out just the people at one table. She was impressed with some divine information. One of the folks at that table was having pain as a result of a bad back problem.

The Lord wanted to heal that person, now, right in the restaurant.

With a sense of awe and trembling, Grace approached the table. She introduced herself to the people and explained why she was there. At first, some looks of disbelief, and then they all pointed to one gentleman seated with them.

He was the one! He had been injured at work and had back trouble! And his back was hurting right now! He was quick to respond. He wanted to be rid of the pain!

He asked Grace what she wanted him to do. Grace had him stand up right there in that crowded restaurant. Fear and apprehension gone now. Faith was rising. She did the "total" thing on him.

He was instantly healed. The pain left! She instructed him to try to do what he could not do before. He bent over and touched the floor — and he was touched by the power of God. Nobody objected! Nobody said a word! But they did watch, and they did see!

I keep uppermost in my mind the purpose of healing. Jesus did miracles so people would believe in Him and be saved. It is always a great thrill when people accept Jesus and I have the pleasure of taking them to church and seeing them mature in Him!

Grace knows now that no matter how long she may stay on this earth, she has found what the Holy Spirit wants her to spend her life doing. She has come to know something else. Something that she can tell all her saved friends! If you have been born-again and received the baptism with the Holy Spirit, what Grace is doing is also what our Lord wants *you* to do too!

The Holy Spirit gave Grace a chorus. It is one that every born-again believer should keep on their lips. The words go like this:

"Holy Spirit, dwell in me.

Holy Spirit, flow thru me.

Let your healing power be the one to set your people free.

Place me in the path of people's needs,

For I am willing to be used by thee.

Help me to be obedient to thy Spirit who dwells in me."

Chapter Three

Reinette — The Contract Price Analyst

Reinette was born-again in April of 1982 and received the baptism with the Holy Spirit the following month. Her job at Randolph Air Force Base as a civilian contract price analyst is both interesting and demanding.

When she first heard about this vision of "ordinary" believers going out and laying hands on the sick, she became so excited that she bought her own set of video tapes. Actually she and her roommate, Lynda, had bought the tapes and held their own healing school. As they watched in the privacy of their own home, the vision began to hit home.

Shortly after that, Reinette attended the healing school at Faith Outreach Center with several hundred other believers.

Excited about the possibilities of this kind of life style, she began to ask people at work about back problems. Since back pain was such a common problem among people in our sitting society, she felt sure there should be plenty of candidates at work.

The first one was a co-worker and friend who was suffering from a backache. In keeping with the training she had received, Reinette did the "pelvic thing" on her.

She was instantly healed and the pain left.

Now, when something like that happens to a person, very few are going to keep it a secret.

Reinette's friend was no exception.

Shortly after she was healed (same day), she brought a gentleman friend of hers to see Reinette. He had been injured in an auto accident. The pain was very severe. His entire spine was out of whack. As he was ministered to, he stated that he could feel something "pushing from inside his body, moving his spine back into place". He was instantly healed!

Later that same day, Reinette attended a meeting at work where a special speaker was to be the guest. During the speech, the speaker mentioned the fact that she was experiencing back pain. After so much successful ministry that day, that was a bad admission to make in front of Reinette unless you were ready to be healed!

After the meeting ended, Reinette approached the woman. She plainly told her what was available to her "In the name of Jesus". The woman at once allowed Reinette to minister to her, and, guess what? She was healed!

Since that time, Reinette has developed quite a name around her office. People continue to come, and they continue to be healed!

Chapter Four

Michelle — The High School Student

Things were pretty easy as long as Michelle wasn't attending public school. For some time her mother had home-schooled her. But now it had become necessary for her to start back to public school. Her mind was flooded with questions. Could she maintain her Christian witness? Could she even maintain her Christian attitude? She was about to find out!

Several weeks had gone by and things seemed to be working OK. She had made some new friends, met a lot of new people, and generally was holding her own.

Then it happened! In the school gym! Right in the middle of a volleyball game! The ball was hit with all the power the hitter could muster. Like a white cannonball it zipped through several hands, and hit Jason full force, right in the side of his head! The force knocked him up against the wall, his head making contact with the wall first.

Michelle had seen the whole thing. And now, she saw Jason sitting on the floor holding his head, plainly in pain.

He spoke very clearly, this voice deep down inside her. A voice she had heard before, even at her young age. This voice, the silent voice of the Holy Spirit, instructed her to go immediately and pray for Jason and he would be healed.

"But Lord, I can't do that!" she responded in her mind.

To that, this still small voice of assurance replied, "That's right! But you're not doing the work, *I am!*"

With that answer, Michelle approached Jason and asked him if it would be all right if she asked Jesus to heal him.

"Yes.....*Please!* It can't hurt any more than it's hurting now!" was Jason's reply.

Michelle gently laid her hands on his head and commanded, *"In the name of Jesus I command this swelling to go down and the pain to stop!*" With her co-students watching in awe, all the swelling *and the pain* went away, right then, at once!

Someone else had been watching! Someone not really knowing what was going on! The gym teacher did not like what she saw, nor what she was told had happened. The anger was evident. It was in her eyes and in her voice. "You have no right to do that sort of thing here," she lashed out at Michelle! "You're expressing your 'faith' at school, and besides, we have a school nurse to take care of that type of thing!"

Michelle disagreed! "All I did was pray for him to stop hurting!"

"You have no right to pray at school," the teacher retorted!

But even as they "exchanged views", the Holy Spirit had placed an ambush. The volleyball game was still going on. Suddenly a cry of pain, and the sight of all the players rushing to a fallen form on the floor! The girl had jumped and lost her balance as she came down. Her knee had struck the floor first and her knee had been knocked out of joint. The damage could be seen by anyone looking on because the dislocated knee joint could be plainly seen under the skin.

With an air of arrogance, the gym teacher turned to Michelle. "OK! See if your God is really powerful. Pray for her!"

The first thought to invade Michelle's mind was doubt, then a question, "Oh no! This is all I need! Why?" But again that impression from down deep, "Go!" So she did! She laid her hands on the injured knee. The girl winced in pain. Michelle spoke to the knee! "In Jesus' name I command healing to this knee." *Nothing!* Sweat began to bead on Michelle's forehead.

"Please, Lord!" she cried in her heart. "You didn't bring me to this point for nothing!"

Then with a flash of inspiration she asked Shelly, "Do you believe God can heal you?" Through the tears came a muffled "Yes!"

Now, in Michelle's spirit, she senses the release.

Now with authority she spoke to the knee: *"In the name of Jesus I command this knee and all the bones within that knee to line up, in Jesus' name!"*

The students are watching — waiting!

The gym teacher is watching — waiting!

And there, before their startled eyes, the bones began to move back into place. Among the watchers, some gasps! Someone says, "Jesus"...but this time not as a swear word, but in awe!

Suddenly Shelly begins to scream, *"Thank you Jesus! Thank you Jesus!*

In shock and conditioned unbelief, the gym teacher just stares.

Now things are certainly different for Michelle at public school. Still not sure of what she saw, or just what happened that day, the gym teacher knows what to do when a student is injured in gym class.

Besides, with Michelle and the Lord, all that paper work is eliminated!

Chapter Five

The Problem

It's a problem with which we have all been faced. It operates not only in the spiritual realm, but in every phase of our lives. It's the problem we run into when we make New Year's resolutions. It plagues us when we try to lose weight, quit watching too much television, or when we determine to spend more time in prayer, or in the Word, *or in ministering healing on a continuing basis!*

We can call the problem by several names. We can call it "not following through on a commitment." It can be labeled being undependable, flaky, or just plain ol' lying. However, we are going to call it "cool down".

It happens when we become excited, or inspired, or enthused about doing something. It can be a simple thing such as spending 15 minutes each morning doing a new exercise by which someone claims to have lost 25 pounds in just two weeks. We have all sorts of good intentions. We fully plan on following through. So we begin one morning, full of visions of how we will look with that 25 pounds gone. The first day, we feel good about ourselves. The second and third day we do just like we vowed to do. Then, when the *work* starts — that's just after the novelty wears off — we begin to wonder if this is really what we want to do.

Then, as happens so many times, after a week or so, we have made a mental choice not to follow through with our well-intended plan. Hang on to that phrase "made a mental choice." That will become more and more important as we continue.

Anytime we fail to follow through on a commitment, no matter what area of life it may involve, we have done damage to both our self-image and our credibility in the eyes of our fellow associates. However, when we fail in a commitment made to our Lord Jesus Christ, the effect can be much more devastating. This can happen at any time we decide to change our lives so as to simply obey what the Word of God tells us to do.

We may become convicted when the Word tells us that we should not enter into "coarse joking". *"Let no foul or polluting language, nor evil word, nor unwholesome or worthless talk [ever] come out of your mouth; but only such [speech] as is good and beneficial to the spiritual progress of others, as is fitting to the need and the occasion, that it may be a blessing and give grace (God's favor) to those who hear it"* (Ephesians 4:29 AMP).

Maybe you like a good funny story. There is nothing wrong with "good" humor. But maybe with you it gets out of hand on occasion. So now you are shown through the Word that this should not be, so you determine that it will stop. And it does, for a few days. As long as you are careful and keep your mind on what you are saying you have control. But just as sure as you relax your mind — there you go again.

And on it goes! It seems we spend our entire lives trying to stop doing certain things that we should not do, and trying to start doing other things we know we should.

Let's get very specific with the problem area which we are going to address in this book. I assume, in reading this, that you have been through the Hunter Healing School and/or have been involved in a Healing Explosion.If you are one of the "average" persons who has been thus involved, let me take a few sentences to describe, more or less, what has happened to you.

1. You were told about the Healing School and that you could be taught how to heal the sick as commanded by our Lord in Mark Chapter 16.

2. With a varying degree of interest, excitement, and/or skepticism, you came to the first session.

3. As you viewed the first hour, you became more and more interested. By the time the course was halfway over, you were one more excited believer. You had begun to see that nothing was impossible to you because you believed. You were ready to lay hands on the cracks in the parking lot. When the practice periods began, you really came unwound.

4. By now you have begun to tell your friends and relatives about your newfound ability. Just let any of them mention a pain or sickness. Wham!

You lay hands all over them. And guess what! Most of them experience some measure of healing, some at once and some later.

5. Then at last, it's time for the Healing Explosion. All the classes and last-minute instructions serve to fire you up all the more. When the time of the Healing Explosion finally arrives — man, sickness, the devil, and hell itself had just better watch out.

6. Within yourself you vow that you have found a *way of life*. You feel that laying hands on the sick and seeing them recover, and as a result receiving Jesus Christ as their Lord, will be something you will do for the rest your life. Because it makes you feel so much a part of what the Holy Spirit is doing on the earth, it can only increase in intensity.

7. So now the Healing Explosion is over. The last few days have been so loaded with activity until it will be so nice to just spend some time thinking about all that has happened. You might just spend time quietly reflecting, thinking about the new friends you have

made during all the training. You'll spend time thinking about the Explosion itself. During this time you get the thought that since you have been so busy, this might be a good time to just relax with your family. Surely there couldn't be anything wrong with that.

Problem

You have *begun* to approach candidacy for *"cool down."* This happens when we begin to allow our minds to be drawn back to reflection on the past events. We need to allow the Holy Spirit to lead us on into the continuing ministry life style of the believer.

Please do not misunderstand! There is absolutely nothing wrong with basking in the afterglow of what God has done during these days of glory. We have been training and gaining invaluable experience in ministry. Certainly, we should think back to those we saw healed when we laid our hands on them. We should remember the things we have heard from Charles and Frances.

But if we are not watchful during this

time, the enemy will do some very tricky things. He knows that the longer he can keep us in this position of inactivity the better chance he has of placing within our minds darts that will move us closer and closer to "cool down".

We'll get much more specific on just how this works and how to stop it from happening later. But sufficient for our discussion here is to say that if the devil can hold us here long enough, certain things will happen. He will aid us in our reflection of past events. He will indeed help us to "reason" ourselves into whatever state of spiritual activity we were before we first started the involvement with Charles and Frances Hunter! But you say, "That cannot happen! I will never be the same."

While writing this portion, I had to stop long enough to conduct a session of our "Advanced Healing School." All of the people attending were graduates of the basic Healing School. They had been involved in the Healing Explosion. All are team members in our "On Call" healing ministry. At the end of the session, I asked if there were any who needed ministering to. Several came forward expressing everything from ingrown toenails to head and neck aches. Next, I called on teams to minister to these. I knew that several of these had "cooled down" from the excitement they had displayed several months ago during the peak of our ministry involvement with the Healing School. They had relaxed their activity with the healing ministry.

I noticed two things! One, they were very hesitant to come forward to minister and two, when they did, *very little happened.*

Beloved, when our Lord opens the way for us to become knowledgeable in ministering as He does with the Hunter training, He is serious, whether we are or not. He demands spiritual growth in us and it is displeasing when we relax in our commitment to Him and in our obedience to His command to fulfill the Great Commission".

So as "cool down" begins to overtake us, we will find ourselves sliding backward in our (1) interest in ministering, and (2) our success in those times when we do actually minister.

Why is this? Why do we all have to fight this battle? Common sense would seem to say that once a believer is exposed to this awesome power flowing through him and setting people free from all sorts of illness (and causing so many to turn to faith in Jesus Christ), he would be set on a course from which he would never stray.

But, as we all know, this is just not so. Those in leadership as a Pastor or Outreach Leader will attest to what we have been saying. Many of those who are so excited at first, slowly "cool down" and finally stop ministering to anybody except when the opportunity is so plain that they would be in blatant disobedience not to minister healing.

But, aside from those cases, you never hear from them. One of the strangest things is that even in those cases where they do minister to someone who gets healed, they don't talk much about it. To all outward appearances, they are doing absolutely nothing. Let me also say that even if you are a leader, you have most likely had to battle the same thing in your own life. In all too many cases, pastors and other leaders have gone into "cool down" along with their people.

Let me tell you why I believe this problem is so devastating to the Body of Christ, and why finding the answer and stopping the problem is so very, very important. Jesus said, *"And this gospel of the kingdom will be preached in all the world as a witness to all the nations, and then the end will come"* (Matthew 24:14 NKJV).

For most of us who grew up in a traditional church, we have somehow left that job to the pastors, evangelists, teachers, missionaries, or others. We felt that if we gave our money to send these out, we were doing our part in fulfilling this requirement. I hope you have learned that is wrong.

Let me put it another way. If we leave the fulfilling of that word to revival meetings, church meetings, street meetings, etc., Jesus Christ will never come back! Someone has said that at the rate the earth's population is increasing, as opposed to the number of preachers, missionaries, and evangelists there are, the job is absolutely impossible.

What are we saying? Simply, that if the job gets done (and it will — somehow) then it will be done as a result of rank and file believers doing, *as a way of life,* exactly what has been taught through the Hunters. But, please listen, it will not be done through people going to Healing Explosions and then fading away in their ministering. It will be done only as thousands and hundreds of thousands of these believers develop an intuitive life style of ministering to those around them. That is what this book is all about. That's what the *"fire card"*, "Keep the Fire Burning" is all about.

As the information on just how "cool down" takes place and how to overcome it is given, allow the Holy Spirit to begin to touch your inner man so that you can renew your mind and spend the rest of your life walking as Jesus would have you walk, "Preaching the Gospel, ministering the baptism with the Holy Spirit, casting out demons, and laying hands on the sick and seeing them recover."

A MODERN MOSES' ROD
by Alex Schneider

Even before the great Healing Explosions began, Barb and I would often drive hours to get to a Hunter service. They had taught us how to minister healing, and that was a great opportunity for us to help minister.

Frances had just asked me to minister to all the lower back problems of people seated in the front row of the church. Excitedly I approached the first lady and was somewhat stunned when she said, "You are not going to grow out my legs!" So I went to the next person, quickly grew out her legs and her back was healed. Then on to the next, and the next until I had ministered to five people and all were healed.

Then I felt a tugging on my sleeve and it was the first lady saying, "I am sorry, will you please grow out my legs, too?" And she was healed.

I had not only seen the power of God work in people's back as their arms or legs grew out, but my polio leg, four inches short, had grown out. However, the polio left me with a crooked spine, like the letter "S", and I probably looked to most people like I needed healing more than they did!

When Moses was complaining to God that the Jews needed a sign, God said, *"And you shall take in your hand this rod, with which you shall do the signs"* (Exodus 4:17).

God has brought to this generation a "rod" for us to use — "growing out arms and legs" to demonstrate visibly HIS miracle power. This has been used more as a witness tool than any other miracle in the Body of Christ!

Chapter Six

To The Leaders

I hope you are a leader, or serving in a leadership position because God called you and put you there. One of the most pitiful things I've ever seen is when a man finds himself in the position of pastor or evangelist, or worse yet, in some hostile foreign land, without God having had anything to do with his being there. What frustration that must produce.

I emphasize this, because, even though we face all the problems with spiritual growth that many of those under us face, (even though Satan hits us with a fierceness that he generally doesn't use against those not in spiritual leadership) we still have the responsibility of those under us! This means that as our "charges" get under attack and begin to slip back or "cool down", the job of stopping and reversing this "cool down" and bringing them out of it is ours under the direction and power of the Holy Spirit.

Although the Holy Spirit can and does deal directly with the individual, He has placed us in leadership for a reason. Listen to the way the Amplified Bible states Hebrews 13:17. *"Obey your spiritual leaders and submit to them — continually recognizing their authority over you; for they are constantly keeping watch over your souls and guarding your spiritual welfare, as men who will have to render an account [of their trust]."* I don't know about you, but to me that is an awesome responsibility.

Jesus, our perfect example, laid for us the perfect example of pastorship. I know that you must agree that if He instructed us to operate in a certain way, then it becomes very important that we follow those examples.

Ephesians Chapter 4 gives very explicit instructions concerning the work of church leaders. Here is how the Amplified Bible states it:

"And His gifts were [varied; He Himself appointed and gave men to us,] some to be

apostles (special messengers), some prophets (inspired preachers and expounders), some evangelists (preachers of the Gospel, traveling missionaries), some pastors (shepherds of His flock) and teachers. His intention was the perfecting and the full equipping of the saints (His consecrated people), [that they should do] the work of ministering toward building up Christ's body (the church)" (Ephesians 4:11,12 AMP).

Now, to a great extent, many pastors have not caught the vision of this ministry. The pastors are to train the saints to do the work of the ministry. Here is where we can see the perfect example of this in the ministry of Jesus.

God has give us a simple way to cause the work Jesus left us to do to be successful. If pastors will employ this simple plan, it will cause their church to literally explode in growth!

It is so simple; just listen to the example Jesus gave us:

In the early part of His ministry, Jesus chose twelve men unto whom he would entrust His ministry. He would train them, and show them how to represent Him.

By the time of Luke, chapter nine, this initial training had been accomplished. Now the time had come to send them forth, or try their wings as it were.

"And Jesus called together the twelve apostles, and gave them power and authority over all the demons and to cure diseases. And He sent them out to announce and preach the kingdom of God and bring healing" (Luke 9:1,2 AMP).

Guess what? They were tremendously successful.

The pattern continues: In Luke chapter 10, we see that seventy more followers had been trained. The Word says, *"Now after this the Lord chose and appointed seventy others, and sent them out ahead of Him, two by two, into every town and place where He Himself was about to come (visit)...Whenever you go into a town and they receive and accept and welcome you, eat what is set before you; and heal the sick in it and say to them, The kingdom of God has come close to you"* (Luke 10:1,2,8,9 AMP).

You must see the pattern plainly. First Jesus trained them. I believe he trained them both by visual example and verbal explanation. He showed them how to heal the sick, cast out demons, etc. Then He issued forth the commission and the anointing. In other words, He gave them the instructions.

Then when His personal earthly work was completed, and He was ready to ascend back to His Father's throne, He did something very important. What He did was so important to His work being continued here, that the devil has pulled out all the stops in keeping the church blinded.

So, in Jesus' name, I ask that you see and hear it now!

As He was about to lift off the earth, Jesus gave both the commission and the principle for receiving the anointing so that His followers down through the ages could do just as the twelve and the seventy had done; that is to go forth and represent Him.

In Mark 16:15-18, He gives the commission. He commands that the believers go forth with the message of the Kingdom of God. He tells us that as we go, certain signs should follow us: we will cast out demons, speak in tongues, have the power over and protection from every evil Satan can cast our way, and then lay hands on the sick and see them recover.

In Matthew 28:18-20 (NKJV), *"Then*

Jesus came and spoke to them, saying 'All authority has been given to Me in heaven and on earth. Go therefore and make disciples of all the nations, baptizing them in the name of the Father and of the son and of the Holy Spirit, teaching them to observe all things that I have commanded you;. and lo, I am with you always, even to the end of the age.' Amen."

Beloved leaders, that is our commission, and it is our only commission. We have not been commanded to go build giant church buildings, great organizations, or anything else to the exclusion of this simple plan. It is a simple, uncomplicated plan.

Everything we do must result in this one thing: people coming into God's Kingdom as a result of a message presented with demonstration of power.

Then in Acts 1:8 (quoted from the Amplified Bible), *"But you shall receive power — ability, efficiency and might — when the Holy Spirit has come upon you; and you shall be My witnesses in Jerusalem and all Judea and Samaria and to the ends — the very bounds — of the earth."*

There it is from His very own mouth — the commission and the power.

Yet one thing is missing: the training has not been given. Why? We find the answer in Ephesians 4:11,12 (quote from NAS): *"And He gave some as apostles, and some as prophets, and some as evangelists, and some as pastors and teachers, for the equipping of the saints for the work of service, to the building up of the body of Christ."*

Can you see it now? We as church leaders, whether apostles, prophets, evangelists, pastors, or teachers, are given the responsibility of training those placed in our care to do the work of the ministry to all those hundreds of thousands around the world who have been baptized in the Holy Spirit, thereby receiving the anointing to carry out the ministry of Jesus.

Only a very few have been properly trained in working with the Holy Spirit to release that power.

That is the vision and the drive of Hunter Ministries as they use the video/audio tapes and books training believers through healing schools all over the world, in every nation, every denomination who believe in Jesus and the power of His resurrection, and through the Healing Explosions and the Great Commission Army.

We want to help you leaders in this training of this mighty Army of God so that they can work in the very power of God as they go forth with His message!

Now, in light of the reference in Ephesians chapter 4 of which I made mention at the beginning of this chapter, this is the way I see it, and I believe the way God sees it.

In so many cases, pastors have tried to keep this ministry to themselves. They will have classes on visiting and witnessing, and they really want their people to witness. But it would amaze you at how many are jealous if any of their flock really begins to move in the instructions found in Mark 16:17,18; or is it because they don't know how to do the supernatural themselves? *"My people are destroyed for lack of knowledge. Because you have rejected knowledge, I also will reject you from being My priest"* (Hosea 4:6 NAS).

If only they could catch the vision of what a dynamic ministry they would have if they would just do what the leaders are instructed to do in Ephesians chapter 4. *"Train the saints to do the work of ministering toward building up Christ's Body (the Church)."* Churches that are now struggling to just exist would *explode*.

What about evangelists? In most cases an evangelist comes to a church for a revival, preaches to a house partly filled with believers for several meetings, preaches nothing but salvation messages, telling saved folks how to get saved, takes a love offering and then leaves town. *Not scriptural!* How welcome the evangelist would be if he would spend this time training the members of the church to *go out into their normal lives,* (where they live, work, shop, and have their being) *and speak the message of reconciliation, and heal the sick, cast out demons, etc.* Instead of leaving that church and pastor with a sense of just another meeting, he would leave it a powerhouse.

About a year ago, I was asked to come to a Baptist church in northern Missouri. They were beginning to move in things of the Spirit and wanted to go on. It could have been a traditional "revival". However, all we did was charge the saints concerning ministering the baptism with the Holy Spirit and healing. At the end of four days, most there had formed into teams and were doing the ministering. After a year, the report from the pastor is that the people are still out fulfilling the Great Commission. The fire has not died out!

What about the teacher? If he is a teacher in the five-fold ministry, then he is also commissioned to train up the saints. There are many teachings he should give to mature the saints, but for this end-time harvest he should focus his training to prepare these harvesters and inspire and exalt them to go out for Jesus. This means that he should be working with young anointed teachers and teaching them that God is always ready to "confirm the message by the attesting signs and miracles..." (See Mark 16:20).

Deflecting "cool down" becomes the responsibility of the ones called by God to raise up ministry among those placed under him in the Lord. In that way this glorious message will spread throughout a church's territory in an almost unbelievable way.

I believe that if you as a leader will prayerfully consider the information you will find on these pages and put it into practice, both in your life and encourage your people to do the same, you will find the problem of "cool down" something that will be overcome.

These same guidelines apply to the

apostles and prophets because all of the five-fold ministry are specifically charged to mature and equip ALL the saints.

We must all start emphasizing this all-important part of the Gospel. Jesus came to earth so people would be saved and gave us his master plan with which to accomplish His purpose.

Chapter Seven

To The Believer

When I say "to the believer," I am speaking primarily to those hundreds of thousands of born-again Spirit-filled folks who make up the vast "silent" and, for the most part, "seated" portion of the church. They are the ones who for years have been seated in the churches listening to preaching and teaching and, in all too many cases, not putting much of what they have heard into practice. But now, for many of them, things have begun to change!

Because you have gone through the Hunter Healing School, been involved in a Healing Explosion, you now face the greatest opportunity of your lives. That opportunity being simply to spend the rest of your earthly life developing into what our Lord has commanded us to be. That is to walk through the earth ministering to people in need by casting out demons, laying hands on the sick, showing lost and dying people that they have been reconciled to God (See II Corinthians 5:18,19), and reproducing disciples of Jesus.

I realize that some of you may have been in churches which teach that signs and wonders are no longer for the church. If so, I trust that you have gotten rid of all that bad coaching. I trust that now, as a believer, you know that Mark 16:17,18 is indeed for you. I pray that everyone reading this realizes you have been left on this earth for a primary purpose — to carry out the Great Commission.

I know you understand that you do not have to go to Africa, or Mexico, or any other foreign country in order to carry out Jesus' command to "make disciples". I hope you understand that the Great Commission is carried out by you right where you are. In your job! At the market! At the beauty or barber shop! In parks while you and your family are picnicking! In homes. Wherever you find people you will find opportunity! So here you are, with this glorious new life facing you.

The Healing Explosion is over! Up until then you were given almost constant instruction on what to do next. But what now? Except for whatever program your church might develop to provide new opportunities to minister, you are more or less on your own.

How do you continue?

Where do you find those sick to whom you can minister?

That answer is simple!

Just look around! They're everywhere.

Yes, but how do I minister to them? Do I just walk up and tell them that I would like to lay my hands on them and heal them?

It is the inability to properly answer these questions that leads us to what we call "cool down".

Let me say again that the job of getting this gospel to the entire world can only be done through you. It is a job which our Lord Jesus said must be done before the end comes. Since we know that the end will come because the Bible is replete with statements concerning the return of Jesus Christ and the end of this age, then we can say beyond any doubt that this job of spreading the gospel to the entire world will be done! That being so, you can either be obedient and be a part of it or be disobedient and not be a part of it!

It is imperative to get past the "cool down" stage and get into the position for the Holy Spirit to develop within you this ministry life style about which we are talking. That is what we hope to accomplish through this book and *"fire card"*. But, it will only work if you are willing to pay the price of commitment to faithfully and continually put this information into practice.

Why not determine right now to do your part in preparing yourself to be used by the Holy Spirit to literally change your portion of this world?

Chapter Eight

What Is "Cool Down" and How Does It Work?

At the point of being born-again, most people are victims of *secularized minds*. That means that all their thinking habits are based on what they can see, hear, taste, touch and smell. This problem is compounded in our modern industrialized society. From the time we first began to think and reason, that thinking and reasoning was guided by a western mindset or worldview that was basically secular, materialistic, and rationalistic.

I maintain that a Christian cannot develop a real "intuitive ministry life style" until this type of mindset is altered. Until then, the first thing our minds will do when dealing with something that goes beyond this way of thinking is to reject it, if only for a moment.

What I mean by this is that we can decide to think differently due to periodic conditioning such as the Healing School. However, because we must force ourselves to think in such a radically altered way, as often times is the case where things such as casting out demons and healing the sick are concerned, we very easily slip back into our former way of thinking. I fully realize that when we are asked about our belief in these things, we will defend our stand that we indeed do believe. I agree that we really do believe "in our spirits" when the Holy Spirit lives in us. It is in our minds that the conflict comes, and that is where the renewing must be done.

There certainly are exceptions. I believe Frances Hunter to be one. There seems to have been an instant mental and emotional alteration in her being. I have known of others who experienced this kind of rebirth. But experience also shows that this is not generally the case. I thank God for those who receive this dynamic conversion because they very quickly get on about the

Master's business.

I was born-again when I was nine years old. Up until that time, the worst thing I had done was chew gum in church and hide under the house when I was supposed to be picking cotton. However, as I grew into adulthood, I was taught secular things from nearly every direction. My salvation was primarily for future benefits. In other words, it would keep me out of hell when I died, but it really wouldn't do much for me before then. So my life experience was based on a secular-rationalistic foundation.

After I had surrendered to the ministry in later years, all spiritual truth (with the exception of getting saved so you can go to heaven when you die) was based on a secular basis. The dictionary describes secular as of or pertaining to the temporal rather than to the spiritual. I placed things such as healing, casting out demons, speaking in tongues, prophecy, etc., in the temporary realm. All these had ceased to exist. Putting these things into some past era was comfortable because there I would not have to deal with them. To some extent, most of us have done the same with all those things that cannot be easily explained according to our scientific thinking patterns.

Please understand, I do not say that Spirit-filled believers *say* that, but to varying degrees we do *think it*. If not, why do we get so sweaty and tight when called on to minister healing in a public place where those watching might violently disagree with our stand? It's more than timidity! It's a simple matter that *in our minds we do not fully believe that all this will really work!* So it becomes very easy for the enemy to lead us back into our old ways of keeping quiet when we are "out there." But we are also told that there are things that can be done about this problem.

Again, so that we can stay on track, let's remember that we are dealing specifically with the problem of "cool down." Even more to the point, we are dealing with "cool down" that affects our developing a "ministry life style" following a Healing Explosion.

We have said that our minds are like the light switch that either allows the power flow to the light fixture (our bodies) releasing it into places where the light needs to shine, or it blocks that flow, allowing darkness to prevail. Let's make that switch a dimmer switch. You know what I mean? One

of those switches that has a knob you turn to
make the light dimmer or brighter.

What makes the dimmer work is a thing
called resistance. As the knob is turned
down, the resistance in the wire carrying the
power is increased. This blocks the flow of
power, making the light dim. Point! Resistance for our demonstration can be equated
with lack of faith, or more to the point, just
plain old undisciplined minds.

That's what we're talking about here!
Having our minds "renewed" so as to flow in
agreement with God's purpose.

Remember the stories at the beginning
of this book? They can demonstrate what
we're saying. Remember how Grace caught
the vision of a ministry life style? I'm sure
that Grace had just as much trouble with
mental "distractions" as anyone else. But
she determined to fight against the tempta-
tion to slip back into the old passive life style
which we have all experienced.

Is Grace special? Certainly! But no
more special than you! What God does
through Grace, He desires to do through you.

Remember Reinette Alecozay who
works at one of the Air Force Bases in San
Antonio. She began to put into use just a few

of the principles given in this book. (A few because she started before the completion of the concept.) Result! Ministering to those around her at work has become as natural as breathing. She now has "strangers" coming to her office for ministry.

Al Garcia, the Park Ranger! He caught the vision early. Ministering to those with whom he came in contact soon became "intuitive". He did not have to "psyche" himself up for it. He would just minister wherever the need appeared.

This same life style is for you! It is God's will for you! It can become a part of your very life — a natural thing for you on a consistent basis! But for most of us, however, the old thinking machine needs to be reprogrammed. The Bible calls it "renewed." We need to get outside of ourselves and become "ministry-conscious". This is the only way to be able to consistently work with the Holy Spirit as He moves upon us to impact our portion of this world.

It is very important that you follow the simple 21-day plan we are about to present to you. Change is never easy! It will take commitment, dedication, and determination. But, I assure you it will be worth it. This is not an exercise in mere mind control. It is learning to think in a way which will allow the Holy Spirit to flow God's power through us as we simply develop habits of thinking that are *with* God instead of *against* God!

Chapter Nine

The Plan

We think according to *habits* that have been built into our minds. We are creatures of habit. Have you noticed how prone we are to do things like taking the same route to work every day, brushing our teeth according to a pattern and sitting in a certain place in church? How do these things become so ingrained in us? Why is it that someone can start a habit like turning on the T.V. when they first come into the house, and then for some reason, when they are unable to do so, it almost disrupts their entire evening? The silence can be deadening.

It is because these habits, which are formed by *simple repetition,* can become so deeply ingrained into our thought process that our entire system rebels at the thought of not satisfying that craving. Consider smoking, drinking, and drugs! We're told that the habit first begins in the mind, and then the body takes over. Can you see how, over the years, we have developed certain responses to certain conditions? Consequently, in order to respond differently, *new habits of thinking must be learned!*

When we enter a restaurant, does our thinking habit center on things like where to sit, what to order, and how much to spend? If so, it will be very difficult for the Holy Spirit to get a message to us concerning ministering to someone *unless we reprogram our thinking during those times*.

According to what people who study habitual behavior tell us, it takes about 21 days to break and replace a habit. We won't be able to properly function in God's will if the only time we are alert to needs around us is when we forcibly fix our minds on the subject. We must *renew* our thinking habits so these high priority things become second nature to us. They must be a very part of our being. We must become aware of needs around us in the same way Jesus did. Can you imagine Jesus missing an opportunity to minister to someone because His mind was preoccupied with something else? *No?* Then we have no excuse for that either.

There are many ways to accomplish this *"intuitiveness"*. As demonstrated by the four testimonies previously given, and the hundreds and thousands of cases where people have caught the vision and have developed this ministry life style we are talking about, some just seem to be able to move on into this. But as we can see in a lot of trained healing team members where most activity stops after the initial thrust is over, *they need help in overcoming the "cool down" problem!* With that in mind, we offer the following plan which, if applied, will help bring you into an exciting, "intuitive", life style of ministry.

I can assure you that the desire of the Holy Spirit is to flow through you with God's power to heal, deliver, and save. But He needs you, He needs you *now* — not when you get everything else cleared out of your mind so you can hear. To Him it must be sort of like a foreman giving a worker instructions which need to be acted on at the

The dictionary describes "intuition" as "The act or faculty of knowing without the use of rational processes; immediate cognition." - "Revelation" gifts operate this way!

very moment they are given, and the worker has his ears filled with wax. We must learn to hear and respond instantly! There may be times when this constant awareness can even save our lives.

The *"fire card"*, "Keep the fire burning", is available as a simple training tool to help you avoid *"cool down"* and to keep you active as a disciple of Jesus *daily!*

Most of us don't need complex training courses. The Hunter Healing School is very simple, but if you don't put into practice what you're told, you will not be effective during the Healing Explosion. It's the same here. This is just the continuing phase — the next step. But again, it will only work to the degree that you make up your mind to be consistent in doing the suggested exercises. Only as you act can the Holy Spirit take these simple things and use them to renew your mind so as to cooperate with Him.

The good morning side of the *"fire card"* is designed to help you get started in the morning. However, just saying it one time would probably accomplish nothing. We are not just trying to read a bit of information or encouragement. What we want to do is plant some new thinking habits.

That's why I ask you to say the good morning side faithfully for three weeks. Why three weeks? Two reasons! One, I feel that the Holy Spirit has given that specific time. Two, as I stated before, it supposedly takes three weeks of *repeated action* to build a habit into our minds. I really believe the Holy Spirit is saying that He wants us to build into our minds a habit of being attentive to His voice while at the same time, watching and listening to our surroundings so He can point out situations where ministry is needed. The morning side will help do this through the concept of repetition.

The good night side helps close out the day and prepare us to sleep, while at the same time receiving from the Lord. As we begin to sleep, if our minds are all jumbled up with what we may have seen on T.V., we will be hindered in the ministry of the Holy Spirit during the night. He wants to speak to us in night visions and dreams even as we sleep. These are important ways the Lord teaches and shows us things we need to know. Again, you must use this card for *at least* three weeks for it to have the effect needed.

Next is something that I cannot overemphasize the importance of enough! *In addition to* your regular prayer time, spend *at least* 30 minutes praying in tongues for the purpose of charging your human spirit with power. In I Corinthians 12:4, we're told that the one who speaks in tongues edifies himself. That word edify means to "build up and strengthen". It is a spiritual exercise! Its benefits are spiritual, although it has outworkings into the physical world. I strongly suggest 30 minutes shortly after awaking in the morning, and then falling asleep after saying the good night side and praying in the spirit. *Very important!*

Determine that during this three-week training period you will put yourself into several ministry situations in addition to your normal contacts that are made daily at work and wherever you go. Here are some suggestions: Choose a Saturday and go to a park for a picnic if the weather permits. Instead of just staying to yourself and doing your own thing, walk around and watch people. As you walk, pray in the Spirit. You will be amazed at what the Holy Spirit will show you about the people at whom you're looking, and at the ministry He'll provide.

Can you see what we're trying to say to

you? In this situation, you have deliberately set yourself in a ministry environment. This is an important part of the minister's life. The Holy Spirit desires to condition us so that no matter where we are or what we are doing, this same attention to needs around us, and to the voice of the Lord, is automatic. You might go to a shopping mall. Just walk — even that's good for you. Watch people! Pray! Listen!

You can go to the airport and do the same thing and this is one of the best places to see some of the most interesting people.

Finally, find someone who will team up with you in this time of training. If you teamed up with someone at the Healing Explosion, then he or she would be the logical one. Witnesing will work better with a partner so that you can encourage each other, pray together, and go minister together. Jesus sent teams out two by two (Luke 10:1).

One of the most effective ways I have ever found to open up ministry involves something that is very traditional and very acceptable. The simple act of greeting someone. The dictionary says that handshaking is the grasping of right hands by two people as a gesture of greeting, leave-taking, congratulation, agreement, or the like. It's something that we all do! It is something that is always expected when we make first contact with someone during the day, when we meet someone for the first time, when we depart the company of someone, and on many occasions when we have agreed with someone about a matter of importance. The point is that handshaking is expected and accepted as a traditional act, and can take place many times during the course of a day's activities. And what an opoportunity it offers to open the way for ministry.

But there is a problem! How many times have we greeted an acquaintance for the first time of the day or maybe even for the first time in a long time, and our greeting was very shallow and careless? Maybe all it involved was a casual "Hi there, Joe! How have you been?" And we did not even hear (or maybe care) what Joe's answer was.

Or how many times have we been introduced to someone and we very casually shook hands, mumbled some sort of greeting, many times not even looking at their face, forgot their name even before we released the handshake, and went calmly on about our selfish ways? What opportunities for ministry have been missed by this kind of action. How many times have we greeted people, traditionally asking them how they were doing, and did not even hear their answer. Or if we did, did not allow it to register in our minds, so we walked off without any kind of response.

Let me encourage you to develop an entirely different sort of greeting. First of all, consider every person you greet very important to God. Consider them as a person in need of something from God. It may be healing, re-birth, or just a word of love or encouragement.

Ask God to lead you to those He has prepared for you that day.

Next, conduct your greeting this way. When you take their hand consider yourself "laying hands" on them. Make the contact firm yet not tight enough to hurt their hand. Consciously, and by *faith* release the power of God as contact is made, in the same way you do when ministering in a healing situation.

Next, look squarely into their eyes. This is a very direct form of deep contact with that person. How do you feel when someone looks intently into your eyes? Over the years of ministry I have learned several things from looking into the eyes of people. First of all, if that person has sin in their lives and has any conviction at all about it, they cannot look you in the eye. They will look away or down toward the floor. You can sense that there is need for some sort of ministry. I do not mean natural ministry, but ministry from the Holy Spirit. Even if they cannot look into another person's eyes because of being timid, there is still need of ministry because being shy or timid is not of God and is a sign of deeper problems.

Here is a very important point! Many times a person will forcibly look into another person's eyes to try to hide problems. *Many times* the Holy Spirit will at that time activate the gift of a word of knowledge and show you things that will break the ministry wide open.

I recall on one occasion when I was introduced to a young lady. She tried to look away, then forced herself to look at me. Instantly the Holy Spirit let me know that at the age of 13 she had been molested. Even some of the details were revealed. The girl had tried to push this event out of her mind. Many problems had come into her life and she could not relate to people. She could not keep friends. Because of this small bit of Holy Spirit revealed revelation, she opened up to ministry and was set free.

Back to our suggested way of greeting. While you are looking fully into their eyes (if possible) call them by their name (important) and ask them about their condition. This is really what we are doing when we say something like "How are you today?" The problem is that we usually ask it automatically without really caring what the answer is. But in this new attention to greeting, both our greeting and our response are going to be totally different.

As we greet them, the question we ask becomes extremely important. It is not asked carelessly, but asked with an intensity that demands an answer. I can assure you, when we greet a person with this degree of sincerity they will, in most cases, open up to us with an answer that is a real picture of their situation.

Have you ever noticed a person who is extremely successful in some type of sales or motivational skills? We can learn a lot from the way they greet people. Now, I know that their motive is different than what we are talking about here. They are looking for clients. But isn't that really what we are looking for? They are looking for customers who will respond to what they have to offer them. Don't we also want to locate people who will respond to what we have to offer them — things like deliverance from bondage, healing, or other ministry needs?

Sure it is! All I'm saying is that we must learn to greet people with an intensity that will let them know we are sincere about our interest in them and "how they are doing."

The way we ask the question and how we respond to their reply is very important. Let me describe a possible encounter. See if something like this would fit into your everyday life as you meet and greet people.

James and Andy are seeing each other for the first time in several weeks. James is the one seeking an open door for ministry. Here is the way it might go.

Andy: "James! How are you? It's been a while."

James: "I'm fine, Andy! And it really has been a while!" (Taking a firm grip on Andy's hand and looking him right in the eye) "Andy, how have you been?" (Waits for him to answer. *Very important!)*

Andy: "Oh! Fine I guess!" (This is an answer which is very common and always needs followed up.)

James: "Andy, is your health good?" (Dependent on the answer here, you may need to press for details about his health. If he gives indication that a health problem exists, then something like:

James: "Gee Andy, I'm really sorry to hear that. Would it offend you if the power of Jesus Christ were to heal you of that problem?" (Very important terminology. Don't ask them if you can pray for them. In most cases you will be speaking to the mountain, not praying.) (If Andy indicates no personal problem such as illness or money problems, ask questions about his family such as:)

James: "Well, Andy, how is your wife doing?" (this could open up a whole lot of worms. If his response indicates no problems, continue by asking him about his children, his job, whatever comes to mind. You'll find that very few people will take offense at your genuine interest in them and their family. So press a bit until you locate the reason his initial response was "Oh! Fine, I guess!" which always indicates some sort of need.

ANOTHER WAY TO WITNESS

The Victory Christian Center of Austin, Texas, has a slightly different practical training which has brought tremendous results! In just two Saturday sessions of witnessing in homes and streets by the trained healing teams, 99 people accepted Jesus, and scores were healed and received the baptism with the Holy Spirit.

Good afternoon (morning) — we were wondering if you could help us? (Pause for a second and then say) My name is_____ _____ and we are with _____ _____(name of church) of _____(city) and we are in the neighborhood looking for sick people who need prayer. (Pause).

First Question:

Do you know anybody in the neighborhood who is sick? (Pause and get the address if somewhere else.)

Is there anybody in your home sick?

If there is a sick person in the home, then make the following *statement*.

"We would like to pray for them, would you please take us to them?"

Ask! What is the nature of the illness?

Say — Oh! that's easy...

Then pray according to the instructions in the healing handbook and *believe for miracles*.

If confined to the bed, (per doctor's instructions) do not ask them to get up.

After praying for the sick — give them scriptures so they can keep their healing: Proverbs 4:20-22, Psalm 107:20, Matthew 8:17, I Peter 2:24.

Ask if there is any additional prayer requests.

Before we leave, let me ask you a question.

Do you know about God's free gift of *eternal life* and are you assured if you were to die right now you would go to heaven?

"No" or "not sure."

(What if they say they are Catholic, Baptist, etc?) Ignore and go to the next statement.

Well, I'll tell you how you can know for sure, and it's quite simple.

God loves you so much that he...(Quote John 3:16).

God has already forgiven you. All you have to do is receive what God has already done for you.

When you receive Jesus as your Savior, then God becomes your spiritual Father and you receive the free gift of *eternal life.*

All you have to do to be saved according to the Bible in Romans 10:9 is *if you confess with your mouth...*(Quote Romans 10:9).

You already believe Jesus is the Son of God, right?

And you believe that God raised Jesus from the dead, right?

Then pray this prayer with me. *Please repeat after me.*

"Father God, I believe in my heart that Jesus has been raised from the dead and I confess with my mouth that "Jesus is Lord." Thank you for forgiving me of my sins and thank you for giving me *eternal life.* In Jesus name I pray. Amen."

Assurance scriptures: (Give the new Christian the following verses). John 3:16, 1 John 1:9, II Cor. 5:17, Romans 10:9-10, Acts

16:30-31, Gal. 2:20.

Stay with the new Christian as long as necessary to get him or her reading and confessing the above scriptures.

You should have a witness card on which you record their names, addresses, telephone numbers and any other pertinent information.

If they say they are attending a "live church", urge them to get into a Charismatic or Spirit-filled group so they can grow in Jesus. If they do not attend a church, regardless of their denomination, invite them to your church and offer to pick them up the next Sunday and take them to church. Follow up until you know they are well grounded in your church, or another exciting Spirit-filled church.

Once you have uncovered the need, be extremely sensitive to the leading of the Holy Spirit as to just how to minister. If they give their consent for ministry, then take out all the stops. Do the "TTT" or any part thereof. Forget about the people around you. If he gives you permission to minister in the present setting, then *go for it!*

I can assure you that when the power of

God begins to visibly operate, those around will do one of two things. They'll either get out of there as fast as possible, or they will stay and watch. If they stay and watch, one of several things will happen. They'll watch in silence, or they'll say "Wow! Did you see that," or "I don't believe that," or "Say, I've got this pain right here. Do you suppose you could do anything about that?" At any rate, the results are certainly worth the risks.

What about those situations where there is not a formal introduction or greeting? These are times like when you are buying groceries and have that incidental contact with the cashier. Here again, it's so simple. We just take advantage of a very polite tradition — speaking to people!

How many times have you gone through a checkout station without even speaking to the person at the cash register? I know that on occasion some grouchy Christian might, but surely not you! But on most trips through that line we at least nod a greeting to the person waiting on us. How easy it is to just take that greeting a bit farther. Here again, with a genuine interest in that person, ask them how they are. They will respond with some sort of answer, and many times

that answer will be a cry for help and under-
standing even though it may be somewhat
hidden. Any ministry should be done in a
moment and done quietly. Remember they
are on someone's payroll!

The most powerful motivation for developing these fabulous ways of opening
doors to ministry is simple. Just remember
that *most of the people* with whom you come
in contact each day are on their way to *hell*.
Most of them have physical, emotional, and/
or financial needs. The person to whom you
so carelessly nod at the checkout counter
may have a terminal disease working in his
or her body. They may even be preparing to
leave as soon as they complete waiting on
you to go for radiation treatment. Who
knows? Certainly you don't! God may have
placed you there in front of them for the express purpose of getting them healed, born-
again and filled with the Holy Spirit.

This is a very simple way to be used
mightily in God's plan of reaching the world
with the Great Commission. It is a very natural way because it fits neatly into our life
flow. It is just taking this very simple concept of greeting people as we go about our

daily activities and making it into a very powerful ministry tool. So go for it! I dare you to try it and see how it will change your life!

Learn to follow after the Holy Spirit, developing your own natural way of opening conversations with people. Most of all, you are there to give to them — not for your own glory or purpose. You are there because you *want to help them;* not because you "have to" help them.

We can wrap it all up this way! We all have weak and undisciplined thinking habits. These thinking habits hinder our service to our Lord Jesus and His work. We are told in His Word that we must not think and act as the world does, but that our minds must be renewed. This will allow us to cooperate with the Holy Spirit and allow the power of God to flow freely from our spirits out through our words and hands into a world that desperately needs to experience this touch.

These habits can be replaced with good habits, but we must work at it long enough for our minds to re-program. This is not a worldly type of mind control any more than changing our bad eating habits would be worldly. We have been instructed to care for the "temple of God". If we have bad eating habits, our temple cannot function properly. And it's the same with our minds.

So *let's do it for Jesus!* Step into the most exciting life possible for one who has become a member of God's family — a life of releasing the life of God into the lives of those all around you.

Today is the day of salvation for someone — now is the acceptable time. Jesus said you will receive power *and be* my witness!

Chapter Ten

Suggested Schedule

As you begin, you will find that it will great-ly help if you will make a commitment to fol-low the program to the letter. The Holy Spirit will honor this commitment and will provide the renewing if you will do your part. With that in mind, following is a suggested three week schedule.

1. Determine a day when you will begin. Set as a solemn commitment before the Lord that during those 21 days you are going to give Him every opportunity to do a work in your thin king patterns and in your habit patterns. In prayer, begin the pro-cess by committing your mind to Him and ask Him to take the information and con-fessions from the Word that you will be reading on the card and use it to build

new thought habits into your very being.

2. Set a time for each morning and each evening that you are going to read the *"fire card"*. Allow enough time at each session for praying in the spirit. Don't be forced to hurry through the exercise. That's very important. Even if you must delay on some day so that you aren't forced to hurry, then do so.

3. Expect the Holy Spirit to begin to place opportunities before you during the day, in keeping with the faith statements on the *"fire card"*. Give Him the chance to begin to build within you a renewed mind that is always attentive to the voice of the Spirit concerning the many opportunities around you.

4. As you begin, right at the outset, set plans for at least one special project during the three week period. This can be a trip to the park, the airport, whatever. Just choose someplace where there are lots of people. Again, expect the Holy Spirit to reveal to you some needs that He wants to meet. Don't force the issue. Allow the Holy Spirit to make the opportunities. Your job is to listen, and be ready to respond.

5. Finally, make it a point during the next three weeks to develop a habit of greeting every person with ministry in mind. It's on the *"fire card"*, and you'll begin to find yourself automatically asking the right questions like "how do you feel today", etc. And, when you do — listen to what they say and listen to what the Holy Spirit says. Look for and expect the doors of ministry to open up in many situations.

Chapter Eleven

A Closing Word To All God's Army!

We have an awesome job ahead. Charles and Frances have caught the vision as to what to do to get the individual saints equipped to fulfill the Great Commission. However, they cannot do that work. God is using them to *"equip the saints for the work of the ministry"* (Ephesians 4:12). It is up to us — you and me to *do the work of that ministry!* I can assure you that all of hell's forces are going to try to stop that work.

Can you imagine with me for a moment? Can you in your wildest thoughts conceive the impact on our country when 100,000 believers catch the vision of "as you go, heal the sick, cast out demons, minister reconciliation"? That's only one out of ten people just in San Antonio, Texas. I'm talking about 100,000 for the entire United States. Think what a small percentage that is even of believers who claim to be Spirit-filled. *It is not an unreachable number!* Yet, just that number of *consistent* ministers working on their jobs, at school, in eating places, in parks, and in homes can totally change the face and the direction of America.

How? Because mixed into that number will be doctors who can greatly affect the abortion problem by reaching those doctors who are doing abortions. Included will be lawyers, school teachers, students, factory workers, radio announcers, TV people — folks from all walks of life. They will be affecting all those different areas of influence. Can you see? It is not by "special events" such as crusades, revivals, and meetings that the change will come. It is through people just like you developing this "life style" about which we have been talking.

As you reach out to those "in your world" the change will come. That is how this next great revival will come! Stop reading and just visualize the possibility of what

I'm saying with 100,000 people reaching out
to wherever need arises around them — and
meeting that need through *supernatural
power* in the name of Jesus. Just think of it! I
believe entire cities will come to Christ.

It is said that in many towns in which
Billy Sunday preached, bars would go out of
business, crime would almost stop, and
businesses would start closing their shops
during business hours for prayer meetings.
If that happened when *one man preached* —
what can happen if a number of believers
consistently minister in *demonstration of
power* on a regular basis. That same change
will take place, but it will not stop a few
weeks after the preacher leaves town! It will
grow and continue to grow. Then it will
spread to other surrounding towns. Can you
just imagine?

How can such an *army* come about?
How important is it for this *army* to be
banded together — aware of each other and
what is happening on the other "fronts"?

Leviticus 26:7,8 in the Amplified Bible
says, *"And you shall chase your enemies,
and they shall fall before you by the sword.
Five of you shall chase a hundred, and a
hundred of you shall put ten thousand to*

flight." I believe that principle is still valid for us in the spiritual realm! Using those figures, we see that with a small number like five, each one can chase twenty. However, as the number grows, the "effectiveness" of each one increases. At the larger number of 100 banded together, each individual number grows to 100, or five times more effective. That means that as the *number* of warriors is added, the effectiveness of the individual warrior is *multiplied!*

When a group of believers band together with a oneness of vision, the Spirit of God can do things through them that will impact the entire world.

Listen! If even a small percentage of those who have attended a School of Healing and have been involved in a Healing Explosion will band together with a common vision (that being to reach those with whom we come in contact every day with the message of reconciliation backed up by *power),* the world will see a demonstration of Jesus Christ which will shake every pagan religion to its very core that has attempted to take up roots in the United States. God can begin to dispel much of the doubt about Christ and His followers. The view the world has about "gentle Jesus, meek and mild" will change. They will begin to see Jesus Christ as the *mighty king of kings* and the head of a *mighty army of demon chasing, disease stopping, overcoming conquerors of whatever gets in our way!*

But it will not happen as long as we are out doing our own little thing and jumping from one "event" to another. We must become single minded! That mind must be to become usable to the Holy Spirit in exactly the way we are talking about here.

I believe the "catalyst" for this Army banding together across the United States can be the *"Great Commission Army"* started by Charles and Frances a few months ago. Through it the "facets" needed for this unifying can become real. For simplicity I'll list them below:

1. A simple "structure" which will cut through all denominational lines to include both pastors and church members in a "communication" relationship not seen before.
2. Representatives who will continue to provide motivation, upgrade training, and encouragement from the Hunter office right on down to the local church and

group level. From there, working through pastors, that motivation will be given to the individual team member. Instead of one church robbing sheep from another, sinners will be added to the Kingdom and the churches.

3. Each member will be supplied with a video tape of the month which will serve a very important function. It will "connect" the individual warrior with the GCA by a message of encouragement from Charles and Frances plus live testimonies of the previous month's seminar, and new teachings. You will also be advised of GCA meetings in your area.

In addition to this, there will be city and area-wide Healing Schools using the six-hour Power Pack video series. This means you can attend a very exciting "refresher" course complete with praise, testimonies, everything, and complete it all in a very pleasant Saturday meeting.

There will also be classes on "How to Operate in the Gifts of the Spirit" available. To be *super effective* in what you will be doing, you need to allow the Holy Spirit to show you things about those to whom you are ministering through the gifts of the

Spirit. There will be classes held to help you in leading a person to faith in Jesus Christ. (This will also be available on audio and video tapes.)

And last, but certainly not least, the GCA member will be involved in something called "Supernatural House Calls". Calls constantly come into the office from cities all over the U.S. People who are sick and need ministry, but do not know who to call. When these calls come in, they will be carried down the GCA line right to you if that person is in your area. You will have the *responsibility* to minister to that person, lead them to Jesus and minister the baptism with the Holy Spirit if need be, and minister healing or whatever else they need and get them into a church where they can grow.

Now, in addition to all this, you will be ministering to those with whom you come into contact each day!

Can you see it now? 100,000 Warriors *actively* being a part of this Army, responding to calls to minister, constantly joining with other Warriors in "upgrade" training, and in encouraging each other. And, in the midst of this, being used to reach people "as they go"?

Thousands of saints are going to be a part of this. Thousands are going to begin to develop this "ministry life style" about which we have been talking! Thousands are going to band together to begin to "capture" our nation and bring it back to its roots — *"In God We Trust"!*

We won't have to try to legislate morality. That is something only the Holy Spirit can place within the fibre of a nation. Once it was there! It can be again! But I believe it will be the result of a grass-roots move of God through people like us ministering "as we go" to *one person at a time,* then sending each new miracle-working disciple out to do the same!

Will you be one of these warriors?

"Go into all the world and preach the gospel to every creature" (Mark 16:15 NKJV).

Go, make disciples!

Supplement

How to Have a Video (or Audio) Healing School

Charles and Frances Hunter have prepared the most effective, the most powerful, the most simple video teaching in the world to train ordinary believers how to do the works Jesus told us to do. In just a few short hours, ordinary Spirit-filled Christians can learn how to heal the sick and actually go about daily ministering healing for the glory of God! The Great Commission is squarely in the hands of BELIEVERS!

These video healing schools are opening all over the world at an unprecedented rate and are changing nominal Christians into giant witnesses!

The end generation is here! We Christians have been chosen to close out this age in preparation for the return of Jesus. Training, maturing, and equipping the saints for the work of the ministry of Jesus is the focus of Jesus for this hour, and the video healing schools are perhaps the most significant tool to accomplish this purpose!

The ministry of a video or audio healing school is endless. First of all, it can bring an excitement and anointing to your people like never before!

It can develop leaders and expand the ministry of your church as those who show a special interest can hold video schools in prayer groups, other churches, etc.

It will reduce the workload of a pastor, because if you give your teams time in services to testify and minister healing, it will bring life to others and to your entire church. Have healing teams minister at every service.

You can hold a monthly miracle service in your own church, or even every Sunday night. Once this is known, it is awesome to discover how many outsiders will come.

Develop leaders who are capable of making "supernatural housecalls" and use them when someone calls in for prayer.

VIDEO HEALING SCHOOL TOOLS

Choose your video series:
HOW TO HEAL THE SICK
"POWER PACK"
Brand new six-hour compacted course
or
Expanded 14 hour series
Two text books: HOW TO HEAL THE SICK
and HANDBOOK FOR HEALING
(Audio tapes may be substituted)

We suggest:
1. Six Hour Power Pack Series:
   Friday night......2 hours
   Saturday............4 hours
        or
   Three nights at 2 hours/night
        or
   All day Saturday
2. Fourteen hour Series:
   2 hours/night, one night/week

CONDUCTING THE SCHOOL

1. Start exactly on time.
2. Show Hour No. 1.
3. Between Hour No. 1 and 2, take offering for the video costs or air-conditioning or other expenses.

4. Allow restroom break and time to purchase books, audio tapes or video tapes.
5. Show Hour No. 2.
6. **Have everyone who has watched the video put into practice what they learned that session. If you do not do this, you will defeat the purpose of the school.**
    THIS IS THE MOST IMPORTANT PART OF THE ENTIRE EVENING.
7. Allow testimony time for students to share what God did through them this session, or since the last session.
8. Repeat the above procedure until all of the hours are viewed and put into practice.
9. At the completion of the school, when each student has viewed all the video or listened to all the audio and studied the books HOW TO HEAL THE SICK and HANDBOOK FOR HEALING, present them with a Certificate of Completion which we will furnish.
    GO MAKE DISCIPLES!!!!!!!!!!!!!!!!

SUPERNATURAL HOUSE CALLS and STREET WITNESSING

There will never be "cool-down" or lack of interest and zeal in the people who continue to let Jesus work miracles through them. Our prime earthly job is to add to the Kingdom and equip and mature the saints. We received power to be witnesses (not just to go witnessing).

Churches and groups should raise up a Great Commission Army of trained believers to reach every person in the city, town, or area where they live. Block off your area on a map and go knock on doors and offer healing, salvation, the baptism with the Holy Spirit, or whatever they need in Jesus. Find ways to have people with needs call and send trained healing teams to minister to them.

One church took their teams out on a Saturday afternoon and won 116 to Jesus, ministered the baptism with the Holy Spirit to about 25; and ministered healing to 25 or 30.

Catch the vision and ministry of Jesus! Develop a life style of witnessing with signs and wonders following every believer and see revival in full bloom!

GO MAKE DISCIPLES!

This teaching is now available in languages of 80% of the world as we go into all the world to preach the Gospel to every creature with signs following. Contact Charles and Frances Hunter for information as to how you may obtain these "supernatural tools" for your missionaries or for your church or group.

Supplement

Great Commission Army
Information

Join
Charles ♥ Frances Hunter's

GREAT COMMISSION ARMY
"Believers fulfilling the Great Commission around the world!"

Join the Great Commission Army today and make healing a life style for the remainder of your life on earth...or until Jesus comes back!

WARNING: DON'T LET "COOL DOWN" ATTACK YOU! (It can be fatal)

● The enthusiasm builds through the Schools of Healing. It continues to build...and build...and build...until by the

Healing Explosion we are ready for anything.

● Our excitement is so great that we are ready to lay hands on anything — then the Explosion is over!

● And...if we are not careful, we begin to experience a sense of "finality".

● Now we've said goodbye to our new friends. We leave the Healing Explosion, basking in the "afterglow." Maybe we go home, talk about what happened, then allow our minds to begin to dwell on the many things needed to be done that will "fit" us back into our traditional life.

What we are unconsciously doing is reverting back to the life style we had before the momentum began to build for the Healing Explosion!

We have started to "cool down."

● And - it will only be a few days until we find it harder and harder to remember the "excitement" and "glow" that was present during the days of the Healing Explosion. *We must not allow this to happen!*

We Have Prayed...

We have really prayed about what we can do to help you make healing a life style! It cannot be a one-time thing where we participate in a Healing Explosion and then return to our old life style. We must continue until Jesus returns.

● We are going to make a healing update video tape once every month for members of the Great Commission Army only.

● This will contain new information on healing, interviews with medical doctors, chiropractors and other members of the medical profession, pastors and healing team members to bring you new help and ideas in many areas.

● This will also contain some awesome news from other members of this exciting Army who have written to tell us their successes and how they did it.

● We have many requests from across the nation for qualified individuals to make housecalls to the sick. Our Great Commission Army will spread healing across the nation and we are planning to network the nation with people who are genuinely and intensely interested in biblically ministering healing to the sick.

● When a call comes in from your neighborhood, you will be notified and requested to make a supernatural housecall within 12 hours, if possible.

● You will be called to minister salvation and the baptism with the Holy Spirit. Learn how to do both. Most people know how to lead someone to Jesus, but you will receive the new book HOW TO RECEIVE AND MINISTER THE BAPTISM WITH THE HOLY SPIRIT to help you.

This is our free gift to members of the GCA.

* * * * * * * * *

How can I join Charles and Frances Hunter's GREAT COMMISSION ARMY?

● To be eligible, you must have read the books HOW TO HEAL THE SICK and HANDBOOK FOR HEALING, watched the 6 or the 14 hour series of video (or listened to the 6 or the 14 hours of audio) and participated in a Healing Explosion.

● In the event you have not finished the above, you may still qualify by completing the training as quickly as possible, and then send in your application.

● Fill in the application form and mail with your Registration Fee of $15, then make a commitment to send at least $20 per month to help finance the Great Commission Army around the world.

● As soon as your application for membership in the Great Commission Army is received, and your registration fee is paid, we will mail you a beautiful certificate stating that you are a bonafide member of the Great Commission Army. Your name will be done in calligraphy to enhance your certificate and an official healing team ribbon will be attached. Each certificate will bear the personal signature of Charles and Frances.

● This will be a proud addition to your home after you frame it.

Can I join with a one-time gift?

● Yes, you can have a lifetime membership for $5,000.00. This will entitle you to receive the special monthly video tape which is available only to members of the Great Commission Army.

● You will receive a full set of ALL of our books, plus a 6 hour Power Pack set of How To Heal The Sick video tapes for your own personal use.

● You will also receive future mailings of all kinds, and a free copy of every new book Charles and Frances write. You will get a preview copy before anyone else does! All of this as our appreciation for your lifetime membership.

● As soon as your application for membership in the Great Commission Army is received and your registration fee is paid, we will mail you a beautiful certificate stating that you are a bonafide member of the Great Commission Army. Your name will be done in calligraphy to enhance your certificate and an official healing team ribbon will be attached. Each certificate will bear the personal signature of Charles and Frances.

● This will be a proud addition to your home after you frame it.

Together let's complete the work Jesus assigned to us!

Here are some suggestions we have found to reduce the possibility of "cool down."

● Determine and make a commitment that you will be actively involved in "laying hands on the sick" as long as you are on this earth.

● Do not allow even one day to pass without finding someone to whom you can minister. At your church on Sunday, ask and find out who is not there because of sickness.

● As you go to a restaurant for lunch, dinner or a snack, take a moment before you get out of your car to program your mind to be in a listening and looking mode. Listen for the Holy Spirit to direct you to people who need healing.

● Find at least two other teams with whom you can have a close fellowship.

> MEET TOGETHER!
> PRAY TOGETHER!
> REVIEW THE VIDEO
> TAPES TOGETHER!

● Go on Healing Field Trips to parks, amusement parks, grocery stores, etc. In addition to that, if there is no unified effort in your city to band the healing teams together, then work toward that goal. If there is such an effort, GET INVOLVED!

● Intensify your reading of the Bible, especially the Gospels and the book of Acts.

● Order the inspiring book "HOW TO OVERCOME 'COOL DOWN' AND KEEP THE FIRE BURNING" with the *"fire card"*, by Charles and Frances Hunter and Ralph Turner.

APPLICATION TO JOIN
CHARLES ❧ FRANCES HUNTER'S
GREAT COMMISSION ARMY

*Print your name EXACTLY
as you want it to appear on your certificate.*

Name _____

Partner # _____ Tel. ( ) _____

Address _____

City/State/Zip _____

Where did you attend video training? _____

_____

For which Healing Explosion(s) did you qualify as a Healing
Team member? _____

Would you like to make supernatural housecalls? ☐ Yes ☐ No

Amount Enclosed: Registration Fee   ☐ $15
                  First Month's Support ☐ $20
                  Total   ☐ $35
                  Yearly Member   ☐ $225
                  Lifetime Member   ☐ $5,000

☐ MasterCard ☐ Visa ☐ American Express

_____ Exp. Date _____

*Please cut on the dotted line (or photocopy) or give information above in letter
and return the form to:
Charles ♥ Frances Hunter
201 McClellan Road, Kingwood, TX 77339
(713) 358-7575*

Supernatural Intensive Care Kit

For those in the church or home who are really interested in being real disciples of JESUS CHRIST, and learning everything they can about healing. This kit contains the best of all our teaching on healing.

*Order individual sets or the full kit
at the special price.*

SERIES I - HOW TO HEAL THE SICK (14 Hours)
VIDEO SET NO. 81141/81142

Jesus gave this masterpiece to Charles and Frances for the Body of Christ. "If Charles and Frances can do it, you can do it too!" This two-part series on healing the sick is being used as the primary teaching for the Healing Explosions, currently held around the world.

Video - $175   NOW $99.95   Audio - $59
Video/Audio Study Guide - $10.00

SERIES II - ADVANCED TEACHING (12 Hours)
VIDEO SET NO. 82531/82532

Everyone who has watched the first 14 hour series will want this new and exciting 12 hour video. The last hour is a series of exciting miracles that you can learn to do also!

Video - $150   NOW $90   Audio - $50

SERIES III - LAKELAND, FLORIDA
HEALING EXPLOSION (12 Hours)
VIDEO SET NO. 82471/82472

The excitement and anointing of a live Healing Explosion is captured on video tape at the Lakeland, Florida Healing Explosion. It was one of the wildest ever! You'll see all the ministry, miracles, and moves of God from start to finish! Includes all training sessions, the Doctors' Panel and the Explosion itself.

Video - $150　　NOW $90　　Audio - $50

SERIES IV - DOCTORS' PANEL (6 Hours)
VIDEO SET NO. 80151

Your healing rate will increase dramatically after you study these wonderful tapes which have been made live at our Doctors' Panels by many different doctors. Study them carefully!

Video - $90　　NOW $49.95　　Audio - $30

HOW TO HEAL THE SICK POWER PACK (6 Hours)
VIDEO SET NO. 80172

Charles and Frances have just completed this super-anointed six-hour version of the HOW TO HEAL THE SICK teaching. Jam-packed with new information, this series also meets the requirements for participation on a Healing Team at the great Healing Explosions! This is not an editing of the 14-hour teaching, this is BRAND NEW!

Video - $100　　NOW $49.95　　Audio - $30
Video/Audio Study Guide $6.00

HOW TO RECEIVE AND MAINTAIN A HEALING (2 Hours)
VIDEO SET 80168

Your healing can become a reality when you learn how to receive it, but to maintain it is a totally different situation. This will give you good advice on how to hang on to what God has given you.

Video - $50　　NOW $29.95　　Audio - $10

*BORN AGAIN, COMMUNION
(No. 80104)
1 Hr.   Charles Hunter

Charles shares what a real born again experience is and what communion actually is. Done live.

Reg. $35   **NOW $19.95**

BRAZIL TOUR 1987
(No. 80257)
1/2 Hour   Charles & Frances Hunter

You will see some of the excitement and miracles that happened when Charles and Frances went to Brazil in 1987. You will feel something you've never felt before. You will love it!

Reg. $25   **NOW $14.95**

COMPEL THEM TO COME
(No. 80106)
1 Hour   Frances Hunter

Compassion for lost souls...a must for every believer.

Reg. $35   **NOW $19.95**

CROSSING OVER (Revised)
(No. 80108)
1 Hour   Frances Hunter

Are you a Mrs. Chocolate Chip Cookie who prefers to stay home or are you a real warrior who prefers to face the Christian battles?

Reg. $35   **NOW $19.95**

DEVIL, YOU CAN'T STEAL WHAT'S MINE
(No. 80175)
1 Hour   Frances Hunter

Know your authority as a believer. Don't let Satan take what is rightfully yours. Fight the battle offensively.

Reg. $35   **NOW $19.95**

DON'T BE A FLAKE
(No. 80110)
1 Hour   Frances Hunter

Sometimes in our zealousness we can be a flake. Flakes need to be instructed and helped so they can become giants for the Lord. LIVE!

Reg. $35   **NOW $19.95**

DON'T PANIC - PRAY
(No. 80174)
1 Hour   Frances Hunter

Did you ever panic when you should have prayed? This is outstanding teaching in this area.

Reg. $35   **NOW $19.95**

*FOLLOW ME
(No. 80112)
4 Hours   Charles Hunter

...Into Abundant Life   ...I Went to Heaven
...Into Life With Jesus   ...Watch Your Language

Charles crashed through the barrier which separates the carnal Christian from the abundant life. His personal testimony will help you to die to self and be set free in Jesus. Baptism with fire!

Reg. $90   **NOW $40**

FORGIVENESS
(No. 80135)
1 Hour   Frances Hunter

A beautiful sharing on forgiveness and what it can do in your life.   Reg. $35   **NOW $19.95**

GET READY
(No. 80157)
1 Hour   Joan Barker

(Charles' & Frances' daughter)

God told Joan to "get ready" and she didn't know for what, but her obedience brought some outstanding results. You will love this.

Reg. $35   **NOW $19.95**

GETTING YOUR ACTS TOGETHER
(No. 81111/81112)
11 Hours   Frances Hunter

The Book of Acts is taught so you will not only learn this vital part of the Bible, but you will also learn to be an active part of the 20th Century book of Acts. This two part series will truly bring the Great Commission down to every day level.

Reg. $150   **NOW $90**
Study Guide also available for $10

GIFTS OF THE SPIRIT
(No. 80258)
6 Hours   Bob Barker

(Charles' & Frances' son-in-law)

Bob Barker is an outstanding teacher in the gifts of the Spirit.   Reg. $90   **NOW $49.95**

GOD HAS EVERYTHING UNDER CONTROL
(No. 80117)
1 Hour   Charles & Frances Hunter
Reminds us who is boss over everything.
                Reg. $35   **NOW $19.95**

*GOD IS FABULOUS
(No. 80118)
2 Hours   Frances Hunter
The story of an "unsaved" Christian who was involved in "churchianity" where thousands of today's Christians live. You will laugh and cry with Frances as she shares her experience of rebirth in Jesus.   Reg. $50   **NOW $29.95**

*GOD'S CONDITIONS FOR PROSPERITY
(No. 80120)
2 Hours   Charles Hunter
Your previous teachings on prosperity will come into focus through this excellent teaching. It will work for YOU!
                Reg. $50   **NOW $29.95**

*GOD'S PART/OUR PART (This Way Up!)
(No. 80121)
3 Hours   Charles & Frances Hunter
For successful Christian living, the believer must do his part. God explains fully which things we must do as well as His part...His promises. Christians must know the rules to fit into His plan for their lives.   Reg. $75   **NOW $35**

HOLY SPIRIT
(No. 80107)
4 Hours   Charles Hunter

This excellent teaching explains very simply who the Holy Spirit is and how He ministers in each individual's life.

Reg. $90   **NOW $40**

HOW TO DEVELOP
THE GIFTS OF THE SPIRIT
(No. 80113)
6 Hours   Charles & Frances Hunter

The gifts of the Spirit are not full-blown when given to us. Outstanding teaching on how all believers can be developed in this area.

Reg. $90   **NOW $49.95**

HOW TO DEVELOP YOUR FAITH
(No. 80116)
1 Hour   Frances Hunter

Having faith is simple when you know how.

Reg.$35   **NOW $19.95**

HOW TO FIND GOD'S WILL
(No. 80136)
2 Hours   Frances Hunter

A simple teaching on knowing the will of God in order to stay within His guidelines and abundant blessings.

Reg. $50   **NOW $29.95**

HOW TO HEAR GOD
(No. 80137)
1 Hour   Charles Hunter

When you learn to hear Him, then all you need to do to operate in faith is to obey Him.

Reg. $35   **NOW $19.95**

HOW TO MAINTAIN DIVINE HEALTH
(No. 80138)
1 Hour   Charles Hunter
God's instructions for health. Reg. $35   **$19.95**

*HOW TO MINISTER THE BAPTISM
(No. 80139)
1 Hour   Charles & Frances Hunter
Every Spirit-filled believer should know how to receive and minister the Baptism with the Holy Spirit. Outstanding! Many are robbed of this beautiful gift because they have not been taught how to receive.   Reg. $35   **NOW $19.95**

HOW TO RECEIVE
AND MAINTAIN A HEALING
(No. 80168)
2 Hours   Charles & Frances Hunter
Bob & Joan Barker
It is important to know how to receive a healing for yourself, and also to know how to teach someone else how to receive a healing! This series by Charles and Frances and Bob and Joan is outstanding because not only does it teach you how to receive — it teaches you how to hold on to what God has given you! Too many people lose their healings because they don't know how to maintain them!
Reg. $50   **NOW $29.95**

*HOW TO RECEIVE THE BAPTISM
(No. 80121)
1 Hour   Charles Hunter
Charles Hunter has led more than a million people into the baptism with the Holy Spirit and speaking in tongues. Simple, easy to understand, scriptural, and SUCCESSFUL.
Reg. $35   **NOW $19.95**

HOW TO WIN SOULS FOR JESUS
(No. 80134)
1 Hour   Charles & Frances Hunter

How you can be an effective soul-winner. Audience participation makes this teaching personal and exciting.

Reg. $35   **NOW $19.95**

INSPIRING YOU OUT OF YOUR SOCKS
(No. 80158)
2 Hours   Charles & Frances Hunter

Do you ever need to be motivated to do beyond what you're doing now? This two-hour tape will inspire YOU two ways. In Abilene, Texas, Charles & Frances asked them to share what happened to them or THROUGH them, and had one of the most inspirational nights of their lives. The second hour will challenge any pastor who wants to be inspired as to what a video healing school can do for his church. It will also stimulate everyone to become vital to their church.

Reg. $50   **NOW $29.95**

JAPANESE EXPLOSION
(No. 80163)
1 Hour   Charles & Frances Hunter

A one-hour live tape from Japan showing the incredible response of the Japanese people to Christianity. You will thrill as you see their aggressiveness in healing the sick, and their hunger to know a living Jesus.

Reg. $35   **NOW $19.95**

LIVING IN THE SUPERNATURAL
(No. 80122)
1 Hour   Frances Hunter

How to maintain a daily walk in the supernatural world of God.   Reg. $35   **$19.95**

MIRACLE SERVICE — VISION OF JESUS
(No. 80123)
1 Hour   Charles & Frances Hunter

The SUPERNATURAL SPREE at Campmeeting '83 is highlighted by the manifested presence of God which was seen in lightning, clouds of glory, angels and great prophecies which came forth. The climax was when Jesus appeared in a bright cloud. Frances tells about this glorious scene from heaven in this tape.   Reg. $35   **NOW $19.95**

NOTHING IS IMPOSSIBLE
(No. 801400
1 Hour   Charles & Frances Hunter

A stirring account of some impossible miracles that will increase your faith.

Reg. $35   **NOW $19.95**

PORTRAIT OF JESUS
(No. 80124)
1 Hour   Charles Hunter

Charles reveals several unique views of Jesus as he paints a spiritual portrait of the Son of God. Extremely anointed.

Reg. $35   **NOW $19.95**

*POSSESSING THE MIND OF CHRIST
(No. 80109)
6 Hours   Frances Hunter

Because we possess the mind of Christ at salvation, this teaching gives you the scriptural basis to know exactly how Jesus would and should act through you in all circumstances. One of Frances' best teachings. You, too, possess the mind of Christ. USE IT!   Reg. $90   **NOW $49.95**

POSSESSING THE WORD
(No. 80105)
6 Hours   Frances Hunter

You can read the Word, confess the Word and memorize the Word and still not possess it. You will truly possess the Word after this outstanding teaching from the book of Ephesians.

Reg. $90   **NOW $49.95**

PUBLIC SPEAKING
(No. 80076)
1 Hour   Frances Hunter

Every Christian should know at least a little about public speaking. Frances' tape is hilariously funny as she gives simple instructions to all on what to do and what not to do.   Reg. $35   **NOW $19.95**

RECOGNIZING YOUR POTENTIAL
(No. 80133)
1 Hour   Joan Barker

Have you reached your maximum potential? If not, this tape is a MUST!   Reg. $35   **NOW $19.95**

RIDE THE BIG WAVE
(No. 80125)
1 Hour   Frances Hunter

The current "wave" is always bigger than the last. Stay on top of what God is doing. Don't wash up on the beach with yesterday's wave.

Reg. $35   **NOW $19.95**

SEVEN STEPS TO SUCCESS IN
MINISTERING HEALING BIBLICALLY
(No. 80164)
1 Hour   Frances Hunter

Everyone who is interested in healing the sick needs to listen to these seven practical steps.

Reg. $35   **NOW $19.95**

SHOW YOUR BADGE
(No. 80153)
1 Hour   Charles & Frances Hunter

A new tape showing you the authority of the believer!

Reg. $35   **NOW $19.95**

SLAIN IN THE SPIRIT
(No. 80126)
1 Hour   Charles & Frances Hunter

Explains this phenomena and its purposes.

Reg. $35   **NOW $19.95**

SOLD ON YOUR PRODUCT
(No. 80176)
1 Hour   Frances Hunter

A man recently asked Frances, "Don't you talk about anything except Jesus?" Her answer was, "No, because I'm sold on my product! And my product is Jesus!" A super anointed tape.

Reg. $35   **NOW $19.95**

SO MIGHTILY GREW THE WORD
(No. 80127)
1 Hour   Frances Hunter

Applying the Bible to daily life, let it grow in your Christian walk.   Reg. $35   **NOW $19.95**

START YOUR DAY WITH GOD
(No. 80128)
1 Hour   Frances Hunter

Frances gets you going with God every morning. Begin the day on the right track.

Reg. $35   **NOW $19.95**

*SUPERNATURAL HORIZONS
(No. 80129)
2 Hours   Charles & Frances Hunter

Breaks down the barrier of "God did it yesterday, but He can't do it today." Tells what God is doing in the NOW. Be aware of what is happening in the world!

Reg. $50   **NOW $29.95**

THE CHARGE
(No. 80250)
1/2 Hour   Frances Hunter

This is one of the most anointed presentations you will ever have the opportunity to witness. You will feel as if Jesus Himself is actually speaking to you. Frances presents the last words of Jesus to His beloved disciples before He left this earth. Jesus is still speaking those same words to every believer today.

Reg. $25   **NOW $14.95**

*THE MINISTRY OF HELPS
(No. 80130)
2 Hours   Frances Hunter

Sometimes the greatest ministry to which God ever calls a person is the ministry of helping others. Recommended reading: "USHERING IN HIS EXCELLENCE" by Ron Kite.

Reg. $50   **NOW $29.95**

THE NAME OF JESUS RINGS BELLS
(No. 80167)
1 Hour　　　Frances Hunter

Three-fold tape. The first few minutes are Frances' testimony of how God healed her of a fatal disease. The second portion is Frances' heart-stirring talk on the real power that is in the name of Jesus. When you hear THAT name, it should set off bells in your head. The last portion is daughter Joan ministering on What's Your Excuse? Outstanding. You'll listen to it over and over!

Reg. $35　　**NOW $19.95**

*THE WORD COME ALIVE
(No. 80100)
2 Hours　　　Frances Hunter

This teaching makes the Bible come alive for 20th century living.　　Reg. $50　　**NOW $29.95**

THREE THINGS GOD SAID
(No. 80101)
1 Hour　　　Frances Hunter

God spoke some prophetic things which the entire Body of Christ needs to hear!

Reg. $35　　**NOW $19.95**

22 WARNINGS TO CHRISTIANS
(No. 80131)
1 Hour　　　Frances Hunter

Recognize danger zones and survive.　　Reg. $35　　**NOW $19.95**

WHO AM I IN CHRIST?
(No. 80132)
2 Hours   Frances Hunter

The average church member really needs to understand who they are in Christ, how to have peace and joy as well as speak with authority!

Reg. $50   **NOW $29.95**

---

*Indicates Book Available

BOOKS
BY CHARLES ♥ FRANCES HUNTER

A CONFESSION A DAY
KEEPS THE DEVIL AWAY

An exciting daily devotional with a selected scripture for every day in the year, plus a confession for that day. Each month is on a special subject for you such as FAITH, FEAR, HEALING, etc. Can be used year after year.

ORDER NO. 3022 $5.95

ANGELS ON ASSIGNMENT

The world is fascinated with fiction stories about angels. Read a true story of Gabriel bringing messages from the heart of God! How God cares for families will stir YOUR heart! The two chapters, HE TASTED DEATH and YOU ARE COVERED (ATONEMENT) are worth the price of the book. A never-to-be-forgotten adventure.

ORDER NO. 3021 $5.95

FOLLOW ME
By his own words, Charles was a "dried-up spiritual prune" until he made a total commitment of his life to God, after thirty-one years of church work! The baptism with fire can be yours, too. Today he's a miracle-working disciple! Especially outstanding for men!   **ORDER NO. 3011 $5.95**

GO, MAN, GO!
Frances took off the day she was saved, and went up and down the highway trying to "sell" everyone on Jesus. She hasn't stopped yet. This will challenge you to BE a witness!
                                   ORDER NO. 3018 $4.95

GOD IS FABULOUS
Involved in churchianity, but not Jesus, Frances' personal testimony hits home to a lot of people. The dramatic story of a sinner who turned into a winner as a '49er. (She got saved at that age!)
                                   ORDER NO. 3015 $3.95

GOD'S ANSWER TO FAT...LOOSE IT!
A fabulous book which works if you do what it says to do, but just like the Bible, it doesn't work unless you follow it. A pastor's wife just lost 100 pounds!   **ORDER NO. 3002 $5.95**

GOD'S CONDITIONS FOR PROSPERITY
Prosperity is not solely dependent on money. Charles gives you a roadmap of what "REAL" prosperity is ! Why settle for a counterfeit when you can have the genuine?   **ORDER NO. 3040 $5.95**

HANDBOOK FOR HEALING

This book is a supplement to HOW TO HEAL THE SICK, it is invaluable because it lists common diseases from A-Z and how to minister healing effectively.   **ORDER NO. 3090 $5.95**

HANG LOOSE WITH JESUS

Did you ever see an apple tree, a pear tree or a cherry tree out there in an orchard straining and grunting and groaning all over the place saying, "I'm growing apples" or "I'm growing pears" or "I'm growing cherries?" No, of course, you didn't. They just "Hang Loose with Jesus" and the fruit grows all by itself. Try the same thing yourself!

ORDER NO. 3016 $4.95

HIS POWER THROUGH YOU

If Jesus gave you the pattern, would you follow what He said to do? He gave it, and this exciting book shares what can happen to people when they actually follow His instructions. God wants to use YOU!   **ORDER NO. 3084 $5.95**

HOT LINE TO HEAVEN

When your prayers hit the ceiling and seem to go no further, then you need to read this outstanding book about Frances as a new Christian who learned how to talk to God — and hear Him! She has never stopped!   **ORDER NO. 3017 $3.95**

HOW DO YOU TREAT MY SON JESUS?

Frances asked a man how he operated in such power and his reply was, "I spend twelve hours every day in the Bible!" Frances thought about all of her daily responsibilities and cried out to God, "God give me at least ONE day where I have twelve uninterrupted hours with you!" He answered by sending her on a futile trip where a plane couldn't land, and by the time she returned home, she had her request answered! What God said to her during those twelve hours is recorded in the book HOW DO YOU TREAT MY SON JESUS?

ORDER NO. 3093 $5.95

HOW TO HEAL THE SICK

"My people perish for lack of knowledge!" A simple book of teaching the believers how to minister healing biblically to fulfill the Great Commission of the Bible. Now published in languages so that four of the five billion people on earth can read it and DO it! It works and works like Jesus said it would! **ORDER NO. 3036 $5.95**

HOW TO MAKE YOUR MARRIAGE EXCITING

A book used by many pastors when counseling people before marriage, and lawyers for those who are contemplating divorce. A fascinating story of two people who found how to make and keep a marriage exciting. Theirs has been tested over 20 years!

ORDER NO. 3044 $4.95

IF YOU REALLY LOVE ME

Frances Hunter says: "Millions have prayed a 'sinner's prayer' at one time or another, and many have prayed it a million times and it never seems to work for them and yet it does for others. What makes the difference? Why do some find all the answers and some fail, even though they are apparently earnestly seeking to walk in victory?"

"Remember, the only part of you that can backslide is the part you have not given to God!"

ORDER NO. 3083 $5.95

IMPOSSIBLE MIRACLES

Have you ever put your problems under the heading of impossible? Impossible for God, impossible for man? Remember what is impossible for man is possible with God! This book is full of stories of people who thought their healing was impossible, but found out differently! **ORDER NO. 3007 $5.95**

MEMORIZING MADE EASY

Tips to keep the Sword of the Spirit on the tip of your tongue. It's easy to memorize Scriptures! A 32-page booklet. **ORDER NO. 3034 $1.50**

MY LOVE AFFAIR WITH CHARLES

God spoke to Charles and Frances 1200 miles apart and told them the exact minute, time and place to be married! They missed each other in the airport because they didn't know what the other one looked like, but God did! A story of two lives committed to God and the miracles that happened when they obeyed Him! **ORDER NO. 3045 $4.95**

NUGGETS OF TRUTH

Exactly what the title says — taken from the book of Proverbs! **ORDER NO. 3001 $3.95**

POSSESSING THE MIND OF CHRIST

We actually do possess a portion of the mind of Christ, but we don't always act like it. This book will make it a reality!   **ORDER NO. 3078 $5.95**

PTLA (PRAISE THE LORD ANYWAY)

Frances at her most humorous best! When a stage collapses, you fall through it, your wig comes off and so do your glasses, and you can still say, "PRAISE THE LORD ANYWAY!" You have a story which will bless people forever.

ORDER NO. 3019 $3.95

SINCE JESUS PASSED BY

How did Charles and Frances ever get into the miracle ministry? The exciting story of the birth of what is today a world-wide ministry in miracles started at a Southern Baptist Church in El Paso, Texas. A book to inspire anyone and everyone! Many are healed as they read this "miracle book."

ORDER NO. 3046 $4.95

the fabulous SKINNIE MINNIE RECIPE BOOK

The companion book to the best-selling GOD'S ANSWER TO FAT...LOØSE IT! This book contains a world of exciting recipes for fat and skinny!

ORDER NO. 3008 $5.95

STRENGTH FOR TODAY

The most unusual "Precious Promise Book" on the market today! Completely different, but perfect and inspirational for everyone!

ORDER NO. 3092 $5.95

SUPERNATURAL HORIZONS

One of the most challenging books ever written by Charles and Frances Hunter because it takes the reader into the supernatural world where Christians should live. "As I opened my Bible to where the 23rd Psalm had previously been, the page was absolutely white! There was no printing of any kind on it. Then I saw the finger of God write five words in the brilliant red blood of Jesus Christ across the blank pages in my Bible!" What would that do to you? **ORDER NO. 3075 $5.95**

THE TWO SIDES OF A COIN

Two of the most beloved people in the evangelical world received the baptism with the Holy Spirit. They had all the arguments against it, but in God's most unusual and perfect timing and way, they received and through this book people all over the world have received this powerful gift of God! A story that speaks to everyone! Hilariously funny as well. Top Ten Best Seller. **ORDER NO. 3047 $4.95**

THIS WAY UP

A teaching book on what is our part and what is God's part, because both are necessary. You can live victoriously at all times provided you know your part and God's part of living for Him!
ORDER NO. 3023 $5.95

WHY SHOULD "I" SPEAK IN TONGUES?

If you or any of your friends have ever asked this question, this book has the answers as you read testimonies of Spirit-filled Christians from all different denominations! **ORDER NO. 3003 $5.95**

VIDEO STUDY GUIDE
HOW TO HEAL THE SICK - 14 Hour Video

This special study guide takes questions from the 14-hour video and then gives you the answers directly behind each hour. Wonderful as a refresher course.   **ORDER NO. 3064 $10.00**

VIDEO STUDY GUIDE - THE BOOK OF ACTS

This Study Guide on the book of Acts can transform your life if you listen to the video or audio of this outstanding teaching by Frances on a 20th Century level for those who want to see the book of Acts re-enacted today!   **ORDER NO. 3063 $10.00**

VIDEO STUDY GUIDE
HOW TO HEAL THE SICK
SIX HOUR POWER PACK

Charles and Frances have produced this super-anointed six-hour version of HOW TO HEAL THE SICK teaching. Jam-packed with new information, this series also meets the requirements for participation on a Healing Team at the great Healing Explosions. This is not an edited work on the 14 hours. IT IS ALL BRAND NEW. The answers are immediately behind each hour's questions!

ORDER NO. 3095 $6.00

GIFTS OF THE SPIRIT SYLLABUS

This accompanies Bob Barker's teaching on the Gifts of the Spirit.   **ORDER NO. 3065 $2.50**